The
Jeffrey
Journey

… a family perched on the wings of an angel

Thoughts About The Jeffrey Journey

I read your book in one sitting when it arrived today, and once again I was overwhelmed with feeling and tears in remembering the circumstances which allowed us to meet, and grow close. In pondering the time I was given to know Jeffrey even a little, and you and your entire family, I can only believe that I was well and truly blessed by the good God. As a nurse, I have come in contact with a great many people, and over the years many, if not most fade from memory, but not Jeffrey. I have him pictured clearly in my mind, lying on his pillow in your lap like a precious jewel the first time we met. (The book clearly explains the tiny touch of skepticism I thought I saw in your eyes that day). No wonder! I am sorry you had to once again "lead another pack" with me in it, but maybe you are meant to teach, not just the nuts and bolts of SMA, but through example, the meaning of true love. True love is what I saw, and true love is what I remember. You, your loving and protective husband (so like good St. Joseph), your generous and brave older kids, and the baby who helped everyone (and especially me) become so much more than we might have been without him. I could not know Jeffrey as you did, but I saw the fruits of his short life, and they seem to be without measure.

You will give hope and inspiration to everyone who reads and listens. Your eloquent journaling of your exceptional journey is uplifting, and despite the sad subject, a joyous map to other travelers wending their way. I thank you from the bottom of my heart.

Mary Ward, RN (Jeffrey's hospice nurse)

You've taken one of life's most difficult tasks, woven through it the threads of significance of life in general, generously shared the medical garbage (i.e. doctors' appointments, doctors' opinions, drugs, equipment, insurance, the COST of everything) that is thrown in with the disease (as if the disease isn't enough in itself) and seasoned it with a balanced dose of humor. How none of us cracks up completely and ends up 12 marbles shy of a dozen is beyond me.

I am deeply touched by the courage that Jeffrey displayed through his short life… thank you for sharing Jeffrey with us.

Jim Gaudreau, SMA parent

Your book helped me get through a tough diagnosis. My son, Samuel, is 5 yrs old with SMA type II. The book was given to me as a gift by a close friend. It took me many stages to get enough courage to read—when I got the book, I cried and put it back in the box, then I read the back cover and put it back in the box, then finally after several months—I read your journey. It gave me an inner strength. Thank you for sharing your story—we all still need to get awareness out about this disease. We will find a cure!! Best always to you and your family.

Janet Schoenborn, SMA parent

I don't quite know what to say to you. Thank you doesn't seem to express the depth of my gratitude to you for writing this book and sending it to me. I received the book yesterday. I started reading it late last evening. I just completed it about 15 minutes ago. I couldn't put it down. As I read earlier today, I kept from becoming emotional by focusing on continuing to read the next chapter. However, I had to break and drive my 15 year old daughter to her volunteer job at the hospital. As we drove we listened to JoAnn's beautiful CD. At that point, the tears began and I had a difficult time turning them off. I returned home to complete the book. I wanted to E-mail you immediately but at this point, my emotions were out of control.

I am 50 years old. I began having symptoms when I was about 9 years old. As I read about Jeffrey, I couldn't help but feel guilty. I have enjoyed 49 1/2 more years of life than he was presented with. As I finished Jeffrey's Journey I came to a realization about myself. I have always put thoughts about SMA on the back burner, so to speak. I have been quite involved in other worthy causes but I think I now realize why I have not contributed more effort to SMA awareness. I think it might have been a defense mechanism for me. Getting to know sweet Jeffrey through the pages of your book has helped me realize I must do more. I plan to review the many resource listings you have provided. I will find a connection with one or more of these and begin doing my part. I will also be corresponding with The Oprah Show to encourage an episode dedicated to Jeffrey's Journey and SMA awareness. I will ask friends and family to do the same. As I explained, this will be a new venture for me.

…Thank you again for sharing your deepest thoughts and memories through your book.

Beth Carollo, SMA (self)

…once I had your book in my possession, I just couldn't resist picking it up and reading it… You are an amazing and gifted writer. Knowing how SMA can ravage a family I was not expecting so much humor in the book… I knew that I would cry throughout the book but had no idea that I would laugh so much, too! You did such a fantastic job of letting outsiders see what a family truly has to go through when faced with this horrible disease… I wish I had been able to meet your little Jeffrey.

Shannon Bostrom, SMA aunt

I recently read *The Jeffrey Journey*!!!! Wonderful book. I am not much of a book person but I couldn't put it down once I started. Sorry to say but that is the first book I read cover to cover so that says alot coming from me!!!

Rick Fiedler, SMA parent

The book not only has inspired me but has helped me a great deal in healing. I read it in one night because I couldn't put it down, so now I am rereading different chapters again! It has made me feel human again and helped me feel okay with different feelings that I had, have and am having... especially the whole "am I insane or crazy for even thinking this way?" Along with not bearing to see my baby suffer another minute, there definitely was a sense of relief when she was free from this heart-wrenching disease! It was so good to hear I wasn't alone and to relate exactly to how you were feeling! You have inspired me to continue to work even harder to get the word out about this genetic killer! I often envision your spot up on your mountain with Taylor and Jeffrey running around playing tag!!! Take care and God bless...

Tisha Reagan, SMA 'angel' parent

I just wanted to let you know that I read your book within just a few nights because I couldn't put it down. Thank you so much for having the courage to share your journey with the rest of us. I had often wondered what it must be like to lose a child since it is possible I may go through that experience someday, but that's not something very many people are willing to talk about.

I really enjoyed your sense of humor, and I learned a lot from your story. Thanks again!

Lisa Kay, SMA parent

Just wanted to comment on the Jeffrey CD your mother made. It's beautiful and Nathan loves it! He relaxes to it while resting in his crib and napping. The nurses love it too!

Jennifer Russell, SMA parent

I absolutely love the book! It has been a great source of inspiration for myself and my husband. Thank you from the bottom of my heart for having the courage to share your personal story with the rest of us.

Need to tell you too that the "Jeffrey book" and CD are getting great use at our house. Tessa used to use the CD to go to sleep every noon and every night… Now she gave it to her little brother (Jack-18 months) to use to go to sleep. So twice a day, sometimes more we listen to it.

Lana Weisenberger, SMA parent

I read it this weekend and wanted to let you know how touched and inspired I am by your journey. It sounds as though Jeffrey was indeed an angel sent to earth for only a short time.

Thanks for sharing your story… as someone who works for an organization trying to eradicate diseases like SMA, your story makes me that much more dedicated to MDA's mission to find a cure.

Meg Hodges, Regional Director—MDA

After receiving my copy of *The Jeffrey Journey* I was hesitant to begin reading, fearing that Jeffrey Baldwin's story would bring the raw emotion of daily routine—of my own son's life and death—back to the forefront of my mind (as if it's not always there already).

What I found, instead, was a kindred spirit wrapped in a story that I could not put down! Helen Baldwin's gripping detail of her family's life, passions and tribulations, in the wake of one of the most deadly of diseases, had me turning pages at breakneck speed. I found myself constantly saying, "Just one more chapter." While this may be due to my own personal situation, Helen fluently describes her feelings and makes you feel as if you are participating in every doctor's visit, in every struggling moment, and in every family embrace.

Contrary to my original thoughts, *The Jeffrey Journey* should NOT be read just by SMA parents or immediate families, but also by doctors, friends, politicians and by anyone interested in reading a riveting human interest story...

Jason Amiss, SMA 'angel' parent

The Jeffrey Journey

… a family perched on the wings of an angel

Helen Baldwin

Illustrations by Katie Baldwin*
(*in earlier days!)

Dreams for Jeffrey CD available at thejeffreyjourney.com

MILVERSTEAD PUBLISHING
Philadelphia | Portland

ISBN-13: 978-09842847-3-3

ISBN-10: 0-9842847-3-3

Cover design and book production by Marin Bookworks
www.TheBookDesigner.com

Milverstead Publishing
31 Rampart Drive
Wayne, PA 19087
(484) 653-6205

Visit us on the web!
www.milversteadpublishing.com

Dedicated with love and appreciation
to Randy, Matthew, and Katie,
family, and friends,
and to the memory of our blessed angel, Jeffrey,
and beloved Papa, Elton Derden

I Remember Jeffrey

I remember Jeffrey
by his soft, brown hair
and bright, brown eyes,
His tiny fingers, toes, and nose,
and his silky, soft skin.

I remember Jeffrey
He was always happy,
Smiling all the time.
When he smiled at me
my insides lit up.

I remember Jeffrey
Sometimes I hear his soft cry in the wind at night,
Or maybe it's not wind at all,
It's his angel wings fluttering from heaven.

I remember Jeffrey.

In memory of Jeffrey Thomas Baldwin
by Bethany Derden, age 9 (barely!)
November 11, 1997

The
Jeffrey
Journey

... a family perched on the wings of an angel

This book focuses on our brief earthly time with our third baby, Jeffrey, diagnosed with spinal muscular atrophy (SMA). However, it is hoped that Jeffrey's invincible spirit, grace, and courage, along with the powerful lessons for the rest of the family from this ongoing life chapter, will resonate with any reader.

♥

There was a tiny angel
Who visited for a while
His secret sparkled in his eyes
and lighted up his smile.

There was a tiny angel
Who came to us one day
He kept his wings tucked out of sight
'til t'was time to fly away.

There was a tiny angel
Who blessed us here on Earth
With laughter, love, and tenderness
he charmed us from his birth.

There was a tiny angel
Who heard heaven call him near
So with a sigh he bid goodbye
to those he loved so dear.

excerpt from 'A Tiny Angel'
by Ravelle Whitener
November, 1997

Foreword

In a lifetime, a person crosses paths with hundreds, maybe thousands, of people. The relationships that ensue may last years, or may last only minutes. If one is lucky, a friendship will be born that will survive the test of time.

I guess I drew the long straw.

My friendship with Helen began out of desperation, the kind that comes only from the heart. Our boys, our babies, were fighting an insidious monster called Spinal Muscular Atrophy… Helen's Jeffrey, whose case was more severe and faster-acting, and my Kevin, who continues his daily battle. We clicked instantly, through the miracle of the Internet, and forged a bond that has carried us through the deepest sorrows and the greatest joys that life has to offer. By the time we finally met in person, we had already seen into the depths of each other's souls.

For those of us who have been unwittingly propelled into the world of disabilities—the world where children die—normalcy requires a new definition. Through her writing, Helen allows a rare and incredible glimpse into a normal family thrown into the most abnormal situation of them all.

Helen's poignant memories of Jeffrey, and her ability to so vividly transpose those thoughts onto paper, paint a realistic—and often painful—picture of what it's like for a mother to help her child live and then to make the decision to help him die.

Though she calls it *The Jeffrey Journey*, this book is more than a chronicle of the short life of a precious child. It is the journey of a family faced with a challenge that from the outset seems unconquerable. Helen takes us along as her family meets life's cruelest curves… and survives.

Thankfully, their journey has not yet ended.

Cindy Schaefer

Once Upon a Time...

...when we least expected it, our family was chosen to embark on a relatively brief, life-altering mission.

While we most certainly would never have volunteered for this particular assignment, the incredible journey provided us with an intense barrage of emotional fireworks and self-discoveries.

Throughout the journey, we stumbled along in a bizarre harmony of shock, numbness, disbelief, panic, uncertainty, grief, despair, chaos, ignorance… and compassion, optimism, acceptance, joy, humor, calm, relief, gratitude, and a previously untapped source of inner strength.

We were afforded a prime opportunity to experience unconditional love and fellowship (on both the giving and receiving ends), along with the indescribable, miraculous power of prayer and faith.

These discoveries would not—*could* not—have reached such incomprehensible potential had we not been bumped off our previous familiar path of comfort and satisfaction and ushered down one replete with gut-wrenching unknowns and unanticipated blessings.

We owe our self-awakenings—and much, much more—not only to the Master Planner of this privileged journey, but also to our fearless guide.

His name was Jeffrey.

When God aims us in
a new direction,
we have to let go
of what we've known,
be willing to embrace
the unfamiliar,
and trust that He
will sustain us
on the journey.

Stormie Omartian
<u>Just Enough Light for the Step I'm On</u>

Before the Journey...

Introduction

A miscarriage in the early 1980s afforded my husband, Randy, and me a perfect opportunity to reassess ourselves. Young, sorta smart, and very energetic, we decided to take a rather major plunge.

Following the usual scheme of things whenever our names were attached, our decision to shift gears from our mainstream (i.e., normal) jobs to become teaching parents at a local residential treatment facility for troubled teens almost wrecked the clutch. Before it registered just what we had gotten our industrious selves into, we were playing parent, teacher, nurse, counselor, sleuth, and parole officer day and night to twelve boys. Ages eight to seventeen, our wards were well-versed in emotional disturbance, drug abuse, family problems, legal scrapes... or all of the above. Considering we'd envisioned jumping into parenthood with a compliant little person less than two feet in length and the weight of a big bag of flour, this was a dive into the deep end of the pool, but we were ready and eager for the challenge. Or so we thought... for a few months.

After our two dogs wore out their welcome as involuntary patrol hairballs, Randy and I decided to return to school for teacher certification—Physical Education and Health for him, Special Education for me. Before starting my own certification process, I spent a year substituting in numerous classes with special-needs kids, not only to persuade our financial ends to meet while Randy focused on his certification, but also to make sure that special ed was indeed the field I wanted to pursue on a long-term basis.

While my most-favorite students were those with mental challenges, I was ready and willing to work in all areas of need; in our hometown of Fort Worth, Texas, there were plenty. I quickly became a regular at a school for orthopedically and multi-handicapped children and soon learned why my number was on speed-dial. Many other substitutes bailed as soon as they saw the students' significant physical limitations and imagined their own responsibilities for the day. Or, if they were a bit tougher (or desperate for the pay), they squeaked through the day and just never went back. I would understand some years later why I did.

In 1985, near completion of my own certification/master's process, Randy was offered a football coaching position for the upcoming school year. The job would entail coaching at an exclusive private school under someone he'd enjoyed coaching with before... a nice bonus. The golden carrot was that he wouldn't have to start on the bottom rung of the highly competitive coaching ladder; he'd be starting out as a coordinator.

There was small hiccup in this grand opportunity, however. The job was in Columbia, South Carolina, a wee bit far for a commute from Fort Worth. The thought of moving away from our home state threw life into a slight momentary spin, but we tried to assess the situation in mature fashion. My brother, Paul, and his wife, Jaymie, had survived quite nicely as transplanted Texans in Bristol, Tennessee. In addition, my folks were aiming to become transplants themselves not too far from Paul and Jaymie upon my father's retirement as an elementary school principal. We decided we should at least scope out the scene and see what Columbia was all about... and to see if there really was life outside Texas.

With a generic certification within my grasp, I would be qualified to tackle students with almost any special need. At least that's what they said. I talked to principals at three schools during our early spring visit to Columbia: one school was designated for students with mental handicaps (my preference), one was reserved for those with emotional handicaps, and one was accessible for students with orthopedic and/or multiple handicaps. As I had completed only one class in the last category (with a professor who spent the bulk of class time discussing her own pregnancy), I knew that school—Brockman—would be my third choice.

If I had one.

~

Drooling profusely at Columbia's breathtaking abundance of early spring dogwoods, wisteria, and azaleas, Randy and I decided to accept the challenge of leaving Texas. In May, we returned to our prospective new home state to find a place to live.

On a hot, muggy morning, which we soon learned was Columbia's claim to fame, we began our house-hunting quest with a delightful realtor. Our mission started well, with the exception of his attempts to convert us to boiled peanuts (blech), but it came to an screeching halt when I found myself on a surgical table. My appendix had decided to explode all the way to my toes, apparently rupturing while Randy and I were meandering on the back roads of America on our trek halfway across the country. Thankfully, it had waited until we reached civilization to speak up. By then, though, peritonitis was speaking up as well.

The hospitalization, surgery, and recuperation were uneventful (except for *my* claim to fame of having the worst ruptured appendix the surgeon had ever seen), and I realized that during the entire diagnostic process, I had found an OB/GYN I liked. I decided I'd make an appointment over the Christmas break to see why we hadn't been able to abide by the *go forth and multiply* command (well, at least the multiply part) since the miscarriage a few years before.

~

From the beginning of my teaching stint in August, I was charmed with and in awe of my new charges—orthopedically and multi-handicapped kindergartners (eventually, ages four to eight years) at Brockman School. My lone certification class in the field—and substitute teaching—would have to suffice for my expertise. I anticipated learning at least as much as I was expected to teach, and I was not disappointed.

My class was a charming and diverse group. A few spoke clearly with their Southern drawls, divulging an overabundance of information (personal and otherwise), while one student spoke clearly with nonsensical thoughts. One mimicked what he heard, complete with drawls, twangs, and whines; another communicated with actions only in a perpetual game of Charades. There were those dependent on wheelchairs or walkers, and some who relied solely on their own unsteady gaits to get around. Some were independent with toileting and feeding, some were not. A few were capable of varying degrees of scholastic accomplishments, while others would never be considered academically inclined in the stretch of anyone's imagination. The eclectic personalities and natural ability to transform even the most serious of intentions into a situation comedy (particularly when I was being observed) provided a most endearing and entertaining assignment, with a heavy dose of hard work tossed in for good measure. A terrific assistant named Dorothy and an incredible staff-turned-great-friends made life grand.

It was about to get even better.

~

We escaped the ~~roach~~ rent house we'd been forced to acquire sight unseen, thanks to the appendix episode, and moved into our very own house not long after the school year began. With the house situation settled and our teaching jobs going well, I planned the next move. Over the Christmas break, I would find out why I hadn't been able to conceive after four years of reckless abandonment.

Much to our utter shock, though, by the time the holidays arrived, the need for detective work was rendered unnecessary, replaced instead by the need to find maternity clothes! It must have been the pine pollen.

Or something.

Highly anticipated by both families, our pregnancy went smoothly, as attested by the fifty pounds I packed on with enthusiastic maternal responsibility. Randy and I signed up for Lamaze, walked faithfully, and ate well (one doctor snorted sarcastically, "I can tell."). We were taking better care of ourselves in general than ever before.

On July 18, 1986, we were blessed magnificently with the arrival of Matthew Joseph, a strapping nine-pounder with as much hair as Randy. He was perfect, and as long as there was frequent access to the milking barn, he was a happy camper.

My folks' former identities as JoAnn and Elton had been scrapped in favor of 'Nana' and 'Papa' the summer before with the arrival of Paul and Jaymie's baby, Jonathan. By Matthew's birth, my folks had moved to our neighborhood in Columbia and had the honors of taking care of their local grandbaby while Randy and I continued teaching to finance diapers and footballs. With their house conveniently situated between our house and Brockman, it was easy for me to assume feeding and cuddling duties during my lunch break every day.

After two years at the private school in Columbia, Randy

landed his first head football coaching job at a private school over 50 miles away. The school received accolades at the State House for winning the state championship in both football and baseball, which Randy also coached. It was an exciting year, but in an effort to replace his significant commuting time with Matthew time, he accepted a 3A head football coaching job in Columbia.

On August 19, 1989, just hours after the second season's opening football jamboree, our family was blessed again, expanded by Matthew's fiercely independent, gorgeous little sister, Katherine Randell... Katie. With two perfect children, great jobs, a cozy house near the grandfolks, and a couple of fine canines, our family was complete.

Life was wonderful.

~

By Katie's birth, Matthew was happily enrolled in a morning preschool program. Mom handled Katie duties without hesitation, although it was determined by the end of the first year that our mini dynamo needed to strut her socialization skills with other little people. So off we went to Miss Sue, a loving soul who cared for teachers' children in her home.

That significant transition coincided with my sixth year at Brockman, another major jolt to the status quo. My position there was no longer one of teaching (granted, a term used loosely at times). Instead, it demanded skilled nursing, thanks to the determination of the powers-that-be to mainstream so many of our other, more academically-abled students into regular schools, if not regular classes. Survival demanded the ability to laugh a lot, which I fortunately shared with my energetic, good-natured new assistant, Ruthie. Granted, we had to look in some mighty odd places to snag it at times, but snag it we did.

That year, the roster and its mind-boggling responsibilities would have scared off the faint of heart, but I was too relieved to be afforded the continued convenience and camaraderie at Brockman to notice.

Jarrod*, non-ambulatory, blind, unable to speak, and—to everyone but his mother—presumed deaf for his complete lack of responding, had numerous seizures throughout the day, each one requiring written descriptive notation. Not a picky eater, he ate everything within reach, including an expensive new foam positioning wedge. Our saving grace was that he was unable to see or move beyond his grazing territory, so if Ruthie and I remained alert enough, everything in our sight was safe. When he was not asleep and/or seizuring, he was either hollering loudly or wailing loudly or chewing... something.

Tina* had a trach and required suctioning throughout the day, several times an hour when there was excessive congestion. She couldn't speak but was ambulatory, cheerful, and able to follow some directions well enough to consider putting her on the payroll. She also provided Mary, the school nurse, and me way too much drama one afternoon with a plug in her trach.

Thomas*, our only returnee from the previous year, was a jewel, always striving painfully hard for as much independence as possible amid extensive physical challenges. Despite faltering and barely intelligible speech (having only a hint of a few teeth didn't help), his laugh was infectious and great medicine for our souls!

Felicia* was stunningly beautiful, visually impaired, non-ambulatory, diabetic, and tube-fed. She required a special foul-smelling formula, which she delighted in spilling on herself and the classroom carpet after lunch by popping her feeding tube button open. Every day.

Buster*, nonverbal and generally content in his invitation-only world, was ambulatory only by traversing the furniture backwards like a slinky. Constant physical assistance was required during meal times to prevent his head from landing in his tray. His perpetually blank stare suggested he was fully unimpressed with either our efforts to keep him safe or our creative attempts to keep a toe in the door of the sanity department.

Winston*, ambulatory with the use of a walker, stubborn as three mules, and nonverbal with the exception of a few unidentifiable sounds coming from his rather conical head, was a leader in direction. He was notorious for rhythmically and cheerfully depositing balls of poop down the hall from the cafeteria to our room, just like Hansel and Gretel. Well, almost. He typically whistled a happy tune of sorts while he worked his magic... and we never lost the way to our room.

By all rights, Teddy*, last but not least in this illustrious group, was supposed to have died after birth, which was the doctor's excuse for not mending his broken arm after his arrival. This little guy was two feet of unbending, crossed and/or seemingly reversed limbs, courtesy of severe arthrogryposis, and was topped off by one foot of dreadlocks. Like several of the others, he was tube-fed and unresponsive, with the exception of an occasional eye blink and quiver.

On Valentine's Day, Ruthie and I were greeted with an addition to our class named Lenora*—and, lo and behold, she talked! Her vocabulary was hardly extensive—"I WANNA EAT!" and "TOYEEEEEEEEESSSS!" was the extent of her repertoire—but, oh, we celebrated. We welcomed our new speaker of the house, then we watched, proudly at first, as she removed her shoes... and tried to eat them. And then she removed her socks and tried to eat them, too. By then we realized her M.O., and sure enough, she then scrambled over to the TOYEEEEEEEEESSSS! and proceeded to stuff everything into her mouth. Uh-oh. Another grazer in the class, only this one moved with determination, purpose, and vision, and she was strong and fast.

Ruthie and I grabbed Lenora, ordered more Geritol and Tylenol, and pondered our new addition, who would require a complete set of hands by herself.

And we laughed to keep from crying.

A lot.

~

Randy's frustration that year with some of the headaches of high school coaching and teaching led to another move—this time to Lenoir, North Carolina, where I retired to full-time mama duties and part-time school volunteering as Randy headed down a path unrelated to football until the coaching bug attacked again two years later. He assumed head football duties at a nearby high school, one with the distinction of possessing the longest losing streak in the state. During his assignment there, Katie started kindergarten, Matthew entered third grade, and the football team began masquerading as a serious competitor. Life was looking up once again.

At the beginning of Randy's third year of this coaching stint, my folks, who had moved to Lenoir first, took a major plunge and headed to the mountains of North Carolina to own and operate a bed and breakfast with cabins on the Blue Ridge Parkway. Thanks to the trees' steady growth spurts, the former 'Mountain View' of the lodge's name was history, unless one dared to venture onto the roof (we didn't), but it failed to matter to us. The peace and tranquility was almost overwhelming. The spectacular scenery indigenous to Ashe County quickly lured Randy and me to follow my folks to the area.

We found an old farmhouse situated on almost fifteen acres

with a pond, small creek, and little mountain with breathtaking views. We minimized the fact that we were downsizing from four bathrooms to one, grateful that it had already been added indoors.

One day before we moved in, Randy and I hiked to the top of our new property and spied a barbed-wire fenced area in the middle of a tangled mass of weeds. Our greenhorn mentality deduced that someone must have owned a horse at one time (even though that didn't seem quite right even to us city slickers), but Randy soon spied hints of faded plastic flowers.

Sure enough, on top of our little mountain was an old cemetery with what looked like about twenty residents. A few sites were marked with stones etched crudely with names and dates, others were marked only with stones. We were fascinated with what we saw and immediately began tossing about ideas for converting the area into a memorial garden full of blooming flowers, a memorial plaque, and a white picket fence.

Upon closer inspection, we discovered a grave marked for a five-month old baby. We would discover later that several of the unmarked graves belonged to babies.

We would also learn, in due time, just how that discovery would apply to us.

~

From the very beginning of our shift from minimally sophisticated city bumpkins to rural mountainbillies, our days were filled with adventures Laura Ingalls-style (or, more often, the Ricardos and Mertzes). The night we moved in, Katie lost her first tooth right in the middle of the chaos that pervaded the house, and she expected me to keep up with it. I was thankful that I needed to retrieve it from the garbage only once.

The well water, the most delicious water we'd ever drunk, turned out to be a swimming haven for frogs and salamanders, resulting in our hauling bottled water from the lodge for drinking until we became proud owners of a well a year later. Wimps, yes.

A week after our arrival, a blizzard deposited over two feet of snow, which was then rearranged haphazardly by the brutal wind into monstrous drifts. As gorgeous as the snow was, the resulting loss of power and the wind's vengeance stopped being fun long before the storm wound down. A snow drift blew into the drafty kitchen by way of the ill-fitting back door, and we watched in awe as it didn't melt. Duct tape acquired instant precedence as a staple, and our back door was promptly stuffed with towels and vinyl tablecloths and taped shut. Until spring.

Flying squirrels found their way into our dining room by gnawing perilously close to the electrical wiring, providing a long, harried night of cheap thrills for Randy, Nellie and Duffy (our fur kids), and me, while Matthew and Katie snoozed unwittingly in their beds. Before we could recuperate from that adventure, our two hairballs, friendly retriever combos with newfound rural mountain gusto, introduced themselves in zealous and unfortunate fashion to a new potential pal—a dark one with a big white stripe down his back. We gasped and gagged as they rushed inside, unleashing the odoriferous welcome over every square inch of carpet and as many inches of upholstery as they could reach. Respirators, tomato juice, rubber gloves, and disposable rain suits were added to the list of must-haves. We were learning.

Pipes froze and cracked, lights flickered, the yard full of countless springs became a swamp with the melting of snow and the onslaught of spring rains, and the interior walls shifted with the insane mountain winds. Bizarre cluster flies, lady bugs, obnoxious carpenter bees, and residential bats materialized in alarming numbers, and we discovered that bed bugs were not a figment of imagination.

We loved our new home.

~

A coaching switch coinciding with the move was in order for Randy. His new duties would be at a school that didn't require such a long, treacherous daily drive up and down the mountain, just one sixty miles across it each day. The coaching position seemed to have great potential, a word we came to use frequently when referring to both the lodge and our old house. Its potential, however, was for disaster that would not only set it apart from all previous coaching duties, but also set the stage for a riveting chapter that would change our lives forever.

Meanwhile, back in Lenoir, our former mammoth house with a mortgage payment to match was eventually rented out to a family thrilled with it and eagerly saving money to buy it. It was another disaster in the making, but we were blissfully ignorant, skipping merrily down the path of wacky routine.

And then, bingo.

...God will never call you to do
what he hasn't already done.

Max Lucado
<u>A Gentle Thunder</u>

The Jeffrey Journey...

*The following is an account based on a journal
of sorts scribbled during our Jeffrey days.*

One

When it became obvious in the fall of 1996 that Mother Nature's irritatingly regular monthly visit was overdue, the consideration of why it might be late skimmed naturally and understandably right over the obvious.

Randy's new coaching job held him hostage in more ways than one, and I'd been busy not only with Matthew and Katie and volunteering in their classrooms, but also with the lodge. My parents were the official innkeepers of this hideaway on the spectacular Blue Ridge Parkway, but I pitched in as another willing 'n' able body, cleaning up and out and otherwise trying to help transform the formerly neglected Cinderella into the beauty we knew she was. It was a full-time effort for all.

With no time or energy to spare, a house the size of a large closet, cessation of unnecessary maternity insurance benefits, and an attempt to subsist on a single teacher's pittance, the one item not on anyone's agenda was another baby in this family.

Surely Mother Nature had consulted her calendar and decided—finally—that mine was a body ripe for the rewards of menopause, and She could just scratch me off her list of monthly nagging.

Oh, that Mother Nature—such a kidder.

Such a master of surprise.

Two

I found a doctor advertising baby delivery services and handed over the urine specimen before returning to the waiting room in shock, trying to absorb what I already knew was the reason for my sitting there… and for my mental paralysis.

A baby. At my age? After over 22 years of marriage? How did that happen? I knew how that usually happened, but I didn't know how it could have happened to us at that particular time. Osmosis, perhaps, from from standing too close to Katie's pregnant teacher? That frog water we drank for two days? Too much clean mountain air? The flying squirrels? Heavens.

What in the world were we going to do with a new baby? Without maternity benefits, money, or room at the inn, a stable might look pretty good by the time we had to clear out a spot for this unexpected little bundle. And my lard supply was already substantial. Wherever would I put on the apparently mandatory fifty pounds I'd so easily amassed with each of the other two pregnancies? The image was ripe for a horror movie.

The shock was giving way to a plethora of emotions and considerations when I was called back to the lab. Not only was the lab result positive, said the cheery, *un*pregnant technician, it was positive *fast*, whatever that meant. I didn't think I wanted to know.

Reeling, I sat in the chair for the initial blood donation, while the nurse asked which doctor I wanted to see. I wanted to see no doctor. I wanted to find myself waking up from what was surely nothing more than the ultimate middle-age nightmare.

And yet, there was the beginning of an inner rumbling I attributed to possible excitement. It was probably an upset stomach due to nerves and sheer disbelief and maybe even a touch of morning sickness. As Katie often said, though, *What's the difference?*

We were going to have a baby.

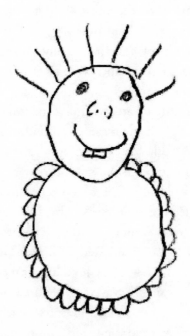

Three

The night of the official word that our family (or, rather I) was expanding was Friday… football night for Randy's high school team. When Matthew, Dad, and I arrived at the stadium during the pre-game stretching routine, I handed a tiny slip of paper to Matthew, the team's ball boy, and he took it to Randy on the field. Matthew had no clue what the '+' on the paper meant, but Randy did, and he still managed to coach the game.

By then I was working up some excitement about another baby and had simply pushed the numerous concerns into the cobwebs of my brain for the time being. It was a joyous occasion, and apparently the good Lord thought we could handle the responsibilities of another baby. We thought we'd done a decent job with the two children we already had, so maybe this unsolicited blessing was our reward!

Goodness knows, we were mature enough in the age category. Some of our peers were already becoming grandparents or at least beginning to deal with college and empty nests.

Well, that day would come for us soon enough.

For now, let the games begin!

Four

Katie's second-grade teacher, starting the school year in a rather pregnant state herself, found it necessary to exit hurriedly from the classroom on more than one occasion. Morning sickness had never been my nemesis during the pregnancies with Matthew and Katie, although I could have hibernated in a heartbeat. Incessant fatigue set in this time, too, no doubt enhanced by the daily madcap chaos of life... and perhaps my rather advanced years.

I kept up with all the usual responsibilities, although I questioned my effectiveness in any of them. Had I not been alerted that the boy I tutored in Katie's class had a fake eye he could pop out with the bat of... well, an eye, I would have been functionally unconscious the first few weeks. The Eye kept me going, at least during my times in her class.

Adding to life's normal buzz, with the lodge and football at the helm, was Katie's enthusiastic participation in gymnastics after school and in evening rehearsals for the local theatre's holiday production, in which she was to be a member of the angel chorus. A packed schedule of late nights fueled my sluggishness even more; the pregnancy itself fueled my need for stretch pants.

It was time to find a tent sale.

Five

When my pudginess had surpassed my usual state of substantial being, Randy and I decided it was time to spring this little matter on Matthew and Katie... and the once-again prospective grandparents, Nana and Papa, and Randy's mom, Nell (alias 'Mamaw'). It would be an entertaining afternoon.

We showed Matthew and Katie the picture of the ultrasound, the only one I'd ever had, and it took Katie, in her almost-seven-and-a-half years of wisdom, a split second to figure it out (although she wrote in the book she began writing later, *We were clueless—what could you expect? We were just kids, not scientists.*). She squealed with delight in circles around big brother Matthew, both literally and figuratively. Our ten year-old firstborn's solitary response—perhaps stemming from a legitimate case of denial—was, simply, "Huh?"

With Katie's boisterous squeals reaching the surrounding counties, we pried Matthew's chin off the floor once he had regained adequate consciousness and then headed to the lodge to tackle my folks.

After ooh-ing and aah-ing over Matthew and Katie's current school pictures, they came across the ultrasound picture and amazingly found nothing odd. "Oh, is this Matthew?" Nope. "Katie?" Uh... nope. "Then who...?" In Matthew-fashion, their bottom lips bungeed to the floor, with Katie still squealing like a pig at the trough.

Life ain't nevur dull in theze heer mowntinz.

We would see to it.

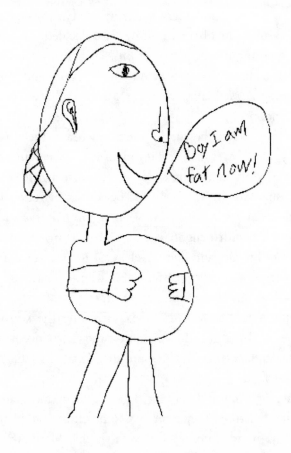

Six

This surprise chapter in our lives started off with unfamiliar ease. Two of the problems, lack of maternity benefits and spare change, were resolved with a state program designed to cover prenatal expenses and first year's medical care for those without insurance, including those (of us) who considered themselves intelligent enough to be prepared for such matters. The lack of insurance coverage was a major concern I could check off the list with great relief.

The lack of space for another family member was optimistically deemed no more than a temporary inconvenience. Randy and I would just set up the crib, the one baby item we had saved for grandchildren, in the corner of our bedroom. We would be walking sideways in our dinky room, but we'd manage. Surely we'd be in a position to add on to the house in a year or so to give us all a bit more breathing room. Words from an optimist.

Gradually, one at a time, we eliminated the most urgent problems. It was really almost too simple, which should have sounded the alarms: *If it sounds too good....*

As the pregnancy progressed, Matthew stayed relatively mum as Katie took full advantage of her keen sense of observation (accompanied by uncanny wit) just as one of the unfriendliest symptoms of pregnancy kicked in. Indigestion. I'd heard after Matthew arrived fully haired that lots of indigestion signaled lots of hair on the baby. That made no sense to me, but I did have indigestion, and we did have beautiful, hairy babies. I figured another hairy little person was on tap this time as well. That or a couple of collies.

Indigestion was legitimately warranted in other areas as well.

The renter family so intent on buying our former house decided to move out unexpectedly instead, leaving us with a cleanup disaster and the whopper of a mortgage payment. Before we could make any attempt to put it back on the market, we would have to fix it up. Again. We could hardly wait, especially since it was an hour's drive away.

In an effort to avoid an imbalance in the Baldwin Department of Catastrophic Situations, we also dealt with eventful circumstances at Randy's school which closely resembled a headhunt. The head in question was Randy's, and we were stupefied as to why it was such a draw. Despite overwhelming favorable support for him from parents and students, the school board voted not to renew his contract, unable to divulge a single explanation for their decision. Even they seemed to wonder what the heck they were doing.

It was a proverbial kick in the seat of the proverbial pants. We failed to identify a single reason why Randy had been targeted for such an absurd attack no one could explain, why he was now no longer in the profession for which he had such passion and talent, why God had allowed such ruthlessness, on top of the house mess, to strike our nice family.

It wouldn't be much longer before we found out.

Seven

Because of my age, advancing at an alarming rate thanks to life's curve balls, my physician, Dr. Kline*, advised me to undergo non-stress tests twice a week during the final few weeks of the pregnancy to make sure everything was still progressing as expected.

The first test proceeded easily and normally. During the second test a few days later, our little bundle with a mind of his own decided to chill out, and the nurse ended up having to prod him out of his doldrums in order to procure a reading.

Prior to the third test, my powerful little charge squirmed and kicked all during our time in the waiting room, but by the time an emergency C-section had been performed (thankfully, not on me), our mini kick-boxer and I were both ready for naps. He decided not to move again until after an hour of my being hooked up to the monitor.

Upon completion of the third test, I waddled over to my scheduled doctor's appointment, at which time Dr. Kline announced he was going to the beach in two weeks and (jokingly) for me not to have the baby until he returned.

Surely he was kidding. There has never been a more enticing invitation for childbirth or other medical urgency than the doctor's being out of pocket, especially when it involves distance. It looked like we'd be having ourselves a May baby, as our little assertion of independence for sure wouldn't hang around until Dr. Kline returned in June. I knew my luck in delivery and in general far too well.

On May 13, the fourth non-stress test went fine. I spent the following school day volunteering in Matthew's class, experiencing enough serious Braxton-Hicks ('practice') contractions and kicking to keep me on full alert. I didn't relish the thought of demonstrating the birthing process at school, most certainly not in Matthew's class. He would have been thoroughly mortified and traumatized for life. Katie, on the other hand, would have beamed with pride, ordering hot water and towels for me and ice cream for the class.

The fifth non-stress test fell on May 15, my 43rd birthday, and our little guy celebrated by doing absolutely nothing. He was again poked and prodded by the nurse, who finally considered herself successful enough in eliciting movement to call it quits. Despite the lack of spontaneous activity, however, my doctor's visit that day turned up some exciting progressive changes, so it looked like we wouldn't be waiting much longer… certainly not until the projected June 1st due date.

Looked like Dr. Kline would be getting a postcard from *us*.

HAPPy Mother's DAY!!

i think the baby is going to weigh 30 pounds maybe? i allso think the baby is going to be a girl, i hope!! the baby will have lots of hair and i know 4 a fact!!!!!!! the baby is going to come on May 31!!

the end!

Love,
katie

Eight

Randy and Matthew went to Lenoir on May 17 to work on the albatross house, while I took charge of getting Katie to her coaches' pitch game. I would have preferred languishing in bed, as my stomach experienced turmoil with a vengeance just before we left, but we managed to arrive at the field mostly intact. I was hardly a model cheerleader mom that day, as I tried in vain to ignore an achy back and rebellious stomach; my sole focus was praying to get through the game and back home to bed uneventfully.

When she saw that I'd packed the car with pillows and the hospital bag *just in case*, Katie asked nonchalantly, "Are you going to have the baby while I'm playing the game?" Jeepers, I hoped not, but I also hoped she wasn't taking any bets.

We did make it back home after the game, and I immediately crawled upstairs to bed and complete inactivity. Katie thoroughly enjoyed unsupervised Barbie activities downstairs that involved a lot of water, and she polished off almost an entire jar of peanut butter effortlessly. I trusted she was safe from harm… or at least any more peanut butter.

The boys arrived home from their own day of fun that evening, and Randy promptly followed me to bed, though not with amorous intentions. He was likewise in a volatile-stomach mode, meaning I would be getting up during the night for whatever needed attention, however many times.

So much for being well-rested for childbirth in my golden years.

Nine

Early Sunday morning, May 18, 1997, the first true-blue contraction hit, two weeks before the due date. At 7am, Randy and I zipped on to the hospital after requesting the sitting services of my folks so Matthew and Katie could remain asleep. We made it to the hospital in record speed, and I waddled with purpose, if not grace, into the emergency room to announce I was there to have a baby. They had probably already figured it out when they felt the floor jar with my entrance.

"When's the due date?" they asked. "June 1," I replied. It was apparent they didn't believe I would be staying, but they humored me and took me upstairs to be checked, anyway. I knew I wouldn't be leaving without a bundle in tow, as my usual doctor was having a vacation at the beach far, far away.

Dr. Brooks*, Dr. Kline's partner and the doctor on call who would be delivering that night, was the one I'd seen only once, of course. Deja vu. The doctor who delivered Matthew was the only one out of a five-doctor practice I'd seen just once, and that had been for the initial consultation. With Katie's no-nonsense arrival, the nurses were pressured to search frantically for an official-looking guy in a white coat to deliver her. Any guy in a white coat, for that matter, as my own doctor piddled at home trying to find the perfect outfit ("You didn't sound on the phone like you were so close to delivery," he said when he showed up, baffled to learn he'd missed the festivities). With Katie, I had to trust that if the one in a white coat delivered bread, maybe he could deliver a baby, too. At least this time, we had a doctor trained in obstetrics. Third time's the charm, or something like that.

After being initially checked and hooked up to everything

imaginable just in case of whatever might go awry, the contractions began in earnest. Whereas Matthew and Katie had popped out with ease, I wondered why the pushes now didn't seem to be getting us anywhere. In actuality, the two or three pushes were serious enough to propel a torpedo across the Atlantic. I sure wouldn't have volunteered to be on the receiving end and hoped Dr. Brooks was ready and well-armed.

At 8:09am, the suspense was over. Jeffrey Thomas Baldwin arrived, looking identical to Matthew, with as much dark hair covering his tiny head as his big siblings had sported. I was able to snuggle and nurse him before he was whisked away for the exams, which revealed, as anticipated, nothing warranting a red flag.

Making his appearance two weeks ahead of schedule, Jeffrey weighed in at just over 7-1/2 pounds and measured 20 inches long. He was the smallest of our three babies but gorgeous.

We transferred without delay into the regular hospital room, occupied by a crowd celebrating the pending dismissal of the new mom assigned to the other bed. Jeffrey was soon brought to me, and he slept... and slept... and slept. I figured the stifling heat of the room was keeping him, like me, in a sedated state, along with the hard work his little body had endured getting him to the real world. He ignored my efforts to nurse him for almost twelve hours, preferring a state of enviable deep sleep. That was something unfamiliar to me, as Matthew and Katie were always ready to nurse from the very beginning.

Randy, always the worrier alert parent, commented on Jeffrey's noticeable abdominal breathing, but as neither the nurses nor the doctor seemed concerned and since he had nursed fine right after his arrival, I ignored his observation with ease and rationalized in my own birthed-out mind that it was due to the early delivery. Jeffrey was going to be a good baby, I could tell, a sign that God knew what He was doing, giving him to a couple not too far away from Senior Citizen discounts.

Life was good. Really good.

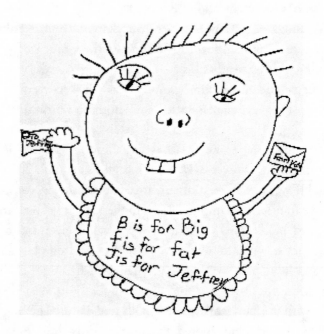

Ten

The afternoon after Jeffrey's birth, Randy arrived at the hospital to chauffeur our new little guy and me home. In the car, I nicked Jeffrey's finger trying to cut his long fingernails, still slightly secured to his fingertips. Welcome home, baby!

We were eagerly greeted in the driveway by impatient big sis, Katie, and Matthew, whose months-long shock instantly shifted into sheer fascination with the details and talents of a newborn. They both held their new baby brother a bit before I fed him, and then we all sat down to our first meal together, courtesy of Randy.

Within five minutes, I somehow spilled ice water on Jeffrey; after the nicked finger episode earlier, it would have been understandable had he begun plotting his escape at that very moment. A quick change into dry clothes and a lot of cuddling calmed him down immediately, though. He was apparently a forgiving soul, which would come in handy. I had a feeling we'd need one in our nutty presence.

As Jeffrey was on my shoulder, he lifted his head, turned it around, and nuzzled for milk. He was strong and owner of a hearty appetite—one of us for sure!

Our first day as a family of five was uneventful, with the exception of Katie's inability to keep her hands off her tiny brother. She picked him up, rocked him, sang and read to him, and tried to get him to take his pacifier. She picked him up when he whimpered and attempted to soothe him herself before reluctantly relinquishing him to me.

Matthew, the ever-cautious soul, allowed me to place Jeffrey in his lap, provided I didn't take more than a step away.

The first few weeks flew quickly. Jeffrey had obviously inherited our families' lust for food after all and merely whimpered for service, even when he legitimately needed prompt attention.

Because he was so undemanding, we could easily tend to the next item of business. Randy's mother, Nell, was due for a two-week visit at the end of the first month, so we organized the troops and cleared out a path to a bed, the fridge, the bathroom, and the comfy chair. I presumed she'd be too busy with the grandkids to notice the generous collection of spiders and webs and bug carcasses all over. Or maybe those would be sufficiently masked by the monster dust bunnies and/or gazillion dog hairs. Thank goodness the kids were cute.

Nell's arrival came the day before I was to undergo removal of a thyroid nodule—one that had ballooned into what felt like a cantaloupe, thanks to the relentless work ethics of the pregnancy hormones. On that day, Randy, Mom, Jeffrey, and I ventured to the hospital thirty-five miles away, while Nell waited at home with Matthew and Katie.

The outpatient procedure went fine. Mom said Jeffrey had been so quiet, it was like he wasn't even there, and he had inhaled his first-ever bottle without a squawk that Mama's milk was in a different container.

We came home a few hours after the surgery, and Jeffrey and I went upstairs to recuperate from our big adventure. He snuggled up, nursed a little, and fell asleep.

Such an easy baby. A perfect baby. A perfect family.

And the fairy tale was slowly coming to an end.

Eleven

Nell's visit was good for all, as she spent almost unlimited time with her grandchildren. On Saturday, July 5, Jeffrey and I stayed home while Randy, Matthew, and Katie drove her to the airport for her return to Texas.

Two days later, I was finally beginning to feel the vague reappearance of a few brain cells and to settle down in some sort of routine when I heard the mail truck drive up.

Matthew and Katie were outside playing with Nellie and Duffy. As I knew they were mastering the all-time favorite country game of Chase the Mailman (the dogs, not the kids), I headed toward the door with intentions of helping contain the hairballs before the mail carrier's departure unleashed the increasingly popular chase opportunity.

I had moved only a few steps toward the door when I heard a sickening thump, followed by screams from both Matthew and Katie. I rushed outside and, to my horror, watched Duffy stagger to the side of the road. He'd been struck by the mail truck, which had then sped away from the scene. I rushed over to Duffy amid screams and tears, watching as he collapsed and rolled down in slow motion into the ditch beside the road.

I slid down and eased him back up to the road, noting in his eyes a peculiar sense of calm. He was in shock. Matthew rushed inside to call a neighbor, as Randy was out on errands; just as the neighbor arrived, though, so did Randy. He carefully placed Duffy into the car and rushed off to the local vet's while I prayed he made it in time.

Back inside the house, I tried to calm Matthew and Katie. By that time, Jeffrey was starving and feeling the tension the rest of us generated, so we all sat down, talked and cried about Duffy and the possible outcomes (there weren't many), and awaited news while I fed Jeffrey. It was a miserable time even for Nellie, who was obviously distraught. She fit right in.

Randy arrived home before too long without Duffy, reporting that the vet would contact us as soon as he could determine anything about his condition. We were staring at what was already on TV—*101 Dalmatians,* of all things—when the phone rang. It was the vet, notifying us that Duffy had not made it. With my big-person rationalization skills, I knew it was probably for the best, but I somehow had to sound convincing to two not-so-big people.

Following the phone call were more tears and questions from Matthew and Katie, all beginning with *Why* or *How come,* and I tried to provide acceptable answers while Randy left to bring Duffy's body home for burial. It was the first time we'd seriously discussed heaven, angels, and God's reason for doing (or allowing) what He did sometimes. The big picture of our life as a family, while never lacking in challenges of one sort or another, had actually been relatively uneventful up to that point, and the topics simply hadn't come up. I was satisfied with how the discussion had gone and how well Matthew and Katie seemed to understand and agree with the big-person rationalization.

Good thing, as it was apparently a rehearsal for something bigger.

Much bigger.

Twelve

Aday or so later, when the tears over Duffy's death had subsided somewhat, my own bizarre months-long fog slowly began dissipating. With lingering effects of Randy's horrendous (former) job situation, lack of gainful employment, and new tenants in our former house contributing only a portion of the mortgage payment each month, I shifted from that end of life's spectrum to the more upbeat happenings in our life. There were plenty: Jeffrey's arrival, Nell's visit, and the end of baseball, coaches' pitch, swimming lessons, and thyroid woes.

I also began taking closer stock of our newest member of the family.

Jeffrey was, unequivocally, as beautiful as Matthew and Katie, and he was certainly an easy baby—he slept and ate, and still only quietly spoke up when he needed something. Anything.

Despite the positive mini evaluation, something nagged at me, something that had probably been stuffed into the darkest crannies of my mind so that I could cope with the rest of life's adventures up to that point. The unidentifiable something that had been hiding in the safety net of the fog, foreign to both of my other pregnancies, was now beginning to demand attention.

It suddenly dawned on me that Jeffrey, just over six weeks old, was seriously lagging in achievements of such physical milestones as holding his head up. Matthew had actually scooted at six weeks, and while I knew that had been an industrious feat, Jeffrey was nowhere near accomplishing even the prerequisites. I realized he hadn't attempted to hold his head up since the post-birth 're-flex' days. I remembered commenting to Dad on the phone that Jeffrey, pushing off my lap with his tiny powerful legs during the conversation, was strong as a horse. What happened?

Instantly, the denial/survival mechanisms began flashing in a dire attempt to push the thoughts—the realization—back into the safety net. *Well, he hasn't had to move, has he? Someone is always holding him, so how could he practice moving?*

Mom said Peggy (her sister) used to sleep all the time as a baby. Peggy, then in her 70s, still taught belly-dancing and water-skiied! *So there,* I theorized to myself, *Jeffrey was no doubt a laid-back soul, right?*

Of course!

That, however, failed to explain his tiny concave chest and the abdominal breathing that had disturbed Randy from the beginning. Both characteristics were impossible to deny and yet had somehow failed to rouse my concern before now. I had simply assumed Jeffrey was another perfect baby, until the awakening only moments before.

Feeling an uncomfortable unraveling of my entire being, I wondered what else I had missed.

Thirteen

My brother, Paul, a doctor, was scheduled to visit with his family (wife Jaymie and children, Jonathan and Bethany) on July 13, which was his birthday. Randy, increasingly alarmed about Jeffrey's abdominal breathing, asked Paul to bring his stethoscope to examine him and to offer his opinion as to what might be the reason.

In a twist of yet-unrecognized irony, the following day, July 14, was to be Jeffrey's two-month well-baby check, but Randy couldn't wait even twenty-four hours longer to find out what was going on. Silently, I knew he was right. Silently, I was petrified.

My stomach was in knots the few days before Paul's arrival. I knew by then that something was seriously wrong and dreaded hearing the words that would label it... and our baby. Drawing on my substitute teaching and Brockman days, my rationalization meter went into overdrive, the memories of various former students flooding into my desperate mind.

Jeffrey possessed a few characteristics of floppy cerebral palsy. *Nah, that student moved, Jeffrey doesn't.* OK, what about arthrogryposis? *Nah, Jeffrey's joints look and feel perfect. Just no movement.* So... how about a combination with, considering our luck, all the most negative aspects of several diseases? It took considerable effort to keep myself from hyperventilating, to rescue myself from the perilous pit of panic.

But I did.

As if under the swoosh of a magician's wand, I automatically morphed into a creative thinking machine, shifting my thoughts from the possible problem to the challenge of a possible solution, beginning mentally to plan a wheelchair-accessible addition to the house. It would not be easy, but we would do it. I firmly believed there was nothing we couldn't deal with. Already, I had diminished the intensity of what might be wrong in an effort to cope. It came in handy to be an optimist!

Optimist? Or master of illusion...

Fourteen

I spent the morning of July 13 on the verge of throwing up. My heart pounded, and I was shaky, chilled, and clammy, despite the fact that it was mid-July and my personal thermostat always threatened to overheat.

We loaded up the essentials—kids, baby, and diapers—and headed to the lodge, with my itchy, swollen, miserable poison-ivy-laden legs and feet from pulling Duffy out of the ditch, a still-tender Frankenstein neck from the thyroid surgery, and an overload of jitters terrorizing my entire body and soul. Paul and his family arrived, and we exchanged the customary chitchat... all on autopilot.

I managed to locate an escape at some point so I could be occupied when Paul went in to examine Jeffrey, napping in the crib. While I would have done anything for Jeffrey, I knew he was in competent hands with Paul, and I knew Randy would ask the right questions... and I didn't think I could talk or even listen without crumbling. Besides, I needed some heavy-duty last-minute, no-holds-barred praying time.

While I submerged myself in folding lodge sheets and towels, Katie came to inform me that Paul was in with Jeffrey. After a few more moments of intense prayer, I somehow made it to the room and opened the door.

Paul reported, with an eerie calm not too unlike Duffy's just days before, that one of Jeffrey's lungs sounded dull, and that there were no reflexes anywhere. None. Jeffrey was a rag doll baby with the frog-legged position typical of floppy babies.

He said that some of the possible explanations for his findings could be serious, and that Jeffrey's doctor would probably

43

want to refer us to a pediatric neurologist as soon as possible. The expression on Paul's face was not comforting, though he tried to scrounge around for a glimmer of optimism to toss into the catastrophe du jour. A glimmer at best.

Somehow my body stayed in a vertical position. With my head and stomach reeling and my heart about to explode, I drifted back into my safety fog for the rest of the day, grabbing any excuse to cuddle Jeffrey and just stare at him as we rocked. Though an optimist by nature, I couldn't stop myself from envisioning all kinds of worst-case scenarios.

I stopped short of envisioning *the* worst.

Fifteen

The day of reckoning finally ended, and I somehow eventually slipped into pretend sleep and a temporary respite from reality. It didn't last long, though, as I bounded up in an impending panic attack to jot down some notes for the doctor. I wondered incredulously how I, who considered myself a loving, attentive, and competent mother, had not heard the warning sirens earlier.

First, the observations of Jeffrey himself:
1. Sleeps a lot & falls asleep pretty quickly when nursing
2. Quiet cry, even when 'demanding' attention
3. Weak cough (which we'd thought was cute!)
4. Lots of yawning (excessive?)
5. A general lack of movement, even during diaper changes
6. No attempt to hold his head up, but does turn it from side to side
7. Chest not growing in proportion to the rest of his body, if at all, even though he's been gaining weight and length well
8. Exceptionally happy and alert when awake.

Next, the odd memories for my own benefit, whatever that might have been:
1. During the pregnancy, I had quit saying, "We just want a healthy baby" in response to "Do ya wanna boy or girl?" for fear Matthew and Katie might think we wouldn't love an 'unhealthy' one. I began replying that we wanted a happy baby, and Jeffrey certainly fit the bill.

2. Thinking of some of the children during my earlier teaching days at Brockman, I had asked Dr. Kline—after a perfectly satisfactory prenatal exam—if babies who didn't move after birth had moved in utero; he said he wasn't sure. Why would I have asked that with Jeffrey, I wondered; I should have thought of it during my pregnancy with Matthew or Katie when I was surrounded at Brockman by children with myriad disabilities, including the inability to move. Jeffrey was moving fine during every exam, with the exception of a couple of sluggish days during the non-stress testing. What made me ask?

3. What was the fog that had kept me in a daze of sorts throughout the entire pregnancy and remained until after Duffy's death and my realization of Jeffrey's delays? I hadn't had more than the usual and expected reduction in mental faculties during the pregnancies with Matthew and Katie. Had it served as some sort of buffer for the challenges we'd faced up to this point? None of the challenges I could even remember seemed worthy of any attention now.

4. During her visit here, Nell received a worrisome phone call that her pregnant granddaughter was undergoing prenatal testing for Down Syndrome. As I particularly enjoyed working with children with Down's, I told her (honestly) that based on my experience and personality, I could handle a child with mental handicaps more easily than a bright child with severe physical limitations. Our own beautiful, alert, 'perfect' baby, whom I had failed to notice wasn't even close to normal physical milestones, lay sleeping nearby.

5. I'd had a bizarre fleeting thought months before that having three children was better than two because if some-

thing happened to one, there would still be two left… almost like an insurance of sorts. The thought was not only bizarre; it was downright creepy to me. Downright unnatural. And I'd considered myself a good mother.

After my frenzied scribbling of notes, a pattern of nauseating evidence emerged, and I went into a certified, full-fledged panic attack.

OH, MY GOD. What if Duffy's death and the opportunity to discuss God, heaven, and angels with Matthew and Katie was just a rehearsal for something bigger?

OH, MY GOD.

Oh, God, no…

Sixteen

I calmed myself down just enough to get ready for the appointment early that morning, and thanks to the escalated sense of urgency, Randy, Jeffrey, and I actually arrived ahead of our scheduled time. I explained to the receptionist that we knew we were early but had something serious going on, that it was no longer a well-baby check. She nodded knowingly and ushered us back to an exam room within minutes.

I withheld from Randy my interpretation of the Duffy event, as there was no need to burden him further with possible speculation. Also, if we were to be seeing another doctor, which I fully anticipated, Randy would need to be focused on the wheel. Any specialist was likely some distance away, and in my present state of mind, I wouldn't be deemed competent enough to get us out of the parking lot.

The nurse weighed and measured Jeffrey, who had continued to grow impressively, and commented that Dr. Brooks would be in soon, that she thought she had just talked to 'your brother.' But of course... Paul. Unbeknownst to us at that time, Paul had searched on the Internet the night before until he located the probable source of the problems with Jeffrey, with brother/uncle emotions intertwining heartbreakingly with physician knowledge. He had thought that because the apparent culprit wasn't a common dilemma, and to save some valuable time for Dr. Brooks, she might appreciate the information he had found. She did appreciate it, though she didn't share with us any of the conversation with Paul, such as his discoveries.

After a brief examination of Jeffrey, which revealed admirable growth but, as we already knew, noteworthy floppiness, zero reflexes, and abdominal breathing, Dr. Brooks left the room to make some phone calls, leaving Randy and me alone with Jeffrey and our rampant imaginations.

She returned to the room after what felt like hours, mentioning a few possibilities of a diagnosis (all of them Greek to us), then referring us to Winston-Salem for consultation with Dr. Smith*, a pediatric neurologist at Bowman-Gray and the first to return her phone call. She initially told us he would see us within the week, but Randy and I both said, NO, we needed to see him that afternoon.

Dr. Brooks agreed (she didn't dare *not*) and told us to go on to Winston-Salem. Because the hospital was almost two hours away, we would be set up for an overnight stay for our convenience. Somehow, the consideration of convenience seemed out of kilter and insignificant to us in the face of such a grim situation, but I was thankful for being looked after by someone who would surely end this nightmare.

Optimism had returned—albeit, briefly—and I began playing the rationalization game again, as if I had ever stopped. *OK... we have a problem, but now we're on our way to learning how to fix it. We have a challenge, but we can handle anything. Wheelchair? No sweat.* My being tossed into teaching orthopedically and multi-handicapped children after a single college course suddenly made sense, and I breathed a sigh of relief. It was beginning to fit, this puzzle we already knew Life was! And perhaps we would even realize the purpose for our new assignment in this lifetime. Jeffrey would be okay, even if it might not be in the traditional sense, and that meant the rest of us would be okay, too!

But not for long.

Seventeen

The ride to Winston-Salem was a somber one, with a barely discernible glint of optimism sequestered in some undisclosed nook in an undisclosed cranny. The only words I spoke aloud to Randy the entire trip were, "Where are we?" and that wasn't until we were almost there.

Words and images flowed silently in my head, though, relentlessly and with overwhelming aplomb. *Jeffrey, Brockman, OT* (occupational therapy), *PT* (physical therapy), *neurological consultation, Jeffrey, wheelchair, Jeffrey, death, Jeffrey, funeral, Jeffrey.* The fiery madness of my poison ivy seared to my bones, and my stomach entertained the thought of super-sized ulcers. Feeling guilty that I had stared at our tiny sleeping prince next to me without speaking, I told him we were going to the big city. He opened his eyes and beamed. Just what did he know?

In due time, we arrived in Winston-Salem, ready to hear some positive news about our little guy. We passed a church with a sign that read, "God's work must be done in God's way." I knew the saying itself was true and timely and targeted our situation, but I didn't know if it could be construed as encouragement... or forewarning.

The first impression of Brenner Children's Hospital, part of Bowman-Gray Hospital, was that it resembled a ritzy hotel, at least to us mountain folks. I trusted they had invested as much in their medical personnel as they had in the design and decor. Randy pulled the car up close to the door so Jeffrey and I could go on inside while he parked.

We didn't have much of a wait after Randy appeared before being called back for the perfunctory information process. Providing vital, accurate info upon request is great fun on a good day and even more so during emotional trauma. The session of names and numbers was a challenge and a blur and a spark for the waterfalls that were sure to gush from my eyes at any moment. No information was easy to recall—not name, rank, or serial number.

Upon completing that part of the admittance process, we were led to our room within minutes. It wasn't overly cozy, but I presumed it didn't matter; we surely wouldn't be staying long.

A pleasant nurse named Barbara came in, jotted down more information, examined Jeffrey briefly, and immediately hooked him up to monitors designed to check heart rate, respiration rate, and oxygen intake. Three electrodes placed on Jeffrey's tiny chest swallowed it completely. Wires were everywhere.

The oxygen intake monitor, placed on Jeffrey's big toe, lighted up with a red glow. In a desperate attempt to find something—*any*thing—amusing or familiar enough to keep us sane for whatever was coming, we dubbed it his 'ET' toe .

ET. Extra Terrified.

Eighteen

Since Bowman-Gray/Brenner Hospital was a teaching facility, small groups of students strolled in and out of our holding tank throughout the afternoon, inspecting their new infant patient from top to bottom and seemingly inside out. Understandably, some parents are adamantly opposed to the constant prodding of their children in such circumstances, but as we were hopeful that maybe one of the wannabe docs just might know or discover something to free us from our private hell, they continued with our blessings. Their quiet demeanor and gentle examination caused no apparent distress to Jeffrey (the pros would take care of that later), and I decided early in this game of horrors that if he could bear being poked and prodded, then we, too, should certainly be tough enough to endure it. We needed answers, and I didn't see how that would be possible without poking and prodding and more poking. Total invasion.

At 7:15pm, five long hours after our admittance, Dr. Smith, the pediatric neurologist-who-knew-all, entered the room to presumably diagnose Jeffrey's problem and, we naively expected, tell us how to address it. He was accompanied by two other official-looking men in white coats, and together they examined Jeffrey, investigating his tongue for fasciculations (quivers, which were present) and holding him prone (on his tummy) and supine (on his back) in the air to test his reflexes. There were none.

Dr. Smith handled Jeffrey as if he were a chicken at the market, but as Jeffrey wasn't fussing and we had to know what was going on, I kept my mouth shut.

After about five minutes of poring over Jeffrey, Dr. Smith

sat down and seemed to ponder momentarily how to handle the presentation of his findings. It didn't take long for him to knock the remainder of our wobbly props away. Far away.

"The probable diagnosis here is spinal muscular atrophy, a disease in which the motor neurons of the spinal cord and brain stem responsible for sending messages to the muscles are affected. The muscles that control movement, sucking, swallowing (pause), and breathing (pause)... will eventually stop functioning.

"There is an option for a respirator. They usually just go to sleep. (*WHAT?*) It is usually peaceful."

WHAT ARE YOU SAYING?

He continued without hesitation. "Jeffrey has a severe case of the most severe type, Werdnig-Hoffmann, or Type 1. There is no treatment or cure. About 80% pass on (*NO!*) by the age of four. (*God, NO!*) It is a recessive genetic condition, which means both of you are carriers. Sometimes I am wrong, but not usually. I don't think I'm wrong now."

In far less time than it takes for me to brush my teeth, Dr. Smith (alias Dr. Doom/Dr. Usually Right), had revealed to us the news that would send us reeling for the duration of our lives. Our baby had a disease we'd never heard of, that we (unwittingly or not) had passed on to him, and which would kill him before kindergarten.

No treatment, no cure, only a waiting game. A game of death. A game I didn't want to play, and neither would anyone else in the family. This medical specialist, who had enlisted in a profession geared toward saving lives, didn't even have the courtesy to tell us the specifics on how long we had before we put our baby in the dirt. No matter that there was probably no way for even Dr Doom/Dr. Usually Right, to know.

Damn him! Damn this disease!

Damn it all!!!!!

In my private twilight zone, I continued rocking Jeffrey in the incredibly uncomfortable rocker in an almost catatonic state, my forgotten poison ivy suddenly revived on a rampage and Dr. Smith's words holding my stomach and head captive in a torturous death vise. My brain thankfully entered the safety of momentary shock, as my heart, completely disintegrating on the spot, was incapable of fully absorbing what we had just heard.

I did ask if my age had anything to do with it (*no*) or if it could have turned up in the prenatal testing, which I had declined as I had with Matthew and Katie (*no, because they wouldn't have known to check for it*). Randy, who was in at least an equal amount of anguish, also managed to ask some questions, but I was too numb for them to register.

Numb was a feeling I'd get to know well. Our baby was going to die, thanks to some savage genes we didn't even know existed, and we didn't know when... or what would come before then.

If the only guarantee in this incredulous situation was death, I would have preferred an instantaneous one.

For me.

Nineteen

The first order of business for Jeffrey that evening, utter devastation or not, was a chest x-ray to see how his lungs looked. His arms were placed and secured above his head, and he was strapped to a board that seemed impossibly narrow. I'd never heard him even cry before, much less howl, but he was quick to voice his misery. I bawled while he wailed. While it lasted only a few minutes, it seemed like days... and it was far from over.

Back in the hospital room, Grand Central Station, commotion was the order of the ~~day~~ night. Blood was drawn from Jeffrey's heels, the beeping machines—irritating and without even an occasional cessation—were checked, his temperature was monitored, and I was told to keep investigating his diapers for whatever treasures he might offer.

Check, check, check.

Beep, beep, beep.

Sob. Pray. Sob.

Chest PT (physiotherapy) was performed every six hours. The pounding on Jeffrey's chest, to keep secretions loosened, was something I had to observe closely in order to be able to do it myself, assuming I wasn't committed to my own ward before we were released.

Still numb to everything but the poison ivy, I rocked and nursed our beautiful, innocent baby whenever possible, wires and all, still trying to grasp and rationalize the whole affair and negotiate tearfully with God. The poison ivy, which had surely reached its excruciatingly intense potential, joined together with this sick twist of fate in making my stomach churn and my head spin (my heart was on its own roller coaster), and we weren't finished in the house of horrors.

The next morning's sun, in all its glory, didn't shed a bit of hope on the situation even for a diehard optimist, and the second day began right back in the torture chambers reserved—in the world of fantasy, anyway—for Dracula, Dr. Jekyll, and Frankenstein.

The painful muscle biopsy to confirm this soul-shattering diagnosis had thankfully been replaced with a relatively new genetic blood test, requiring an amount of blood inadequately provided by the heels. The three nurses, who had never heard of SMA, much less the blood test, had to find another spot, one that hadn't yet been tapped.

Their reluctant decision and, realistically, probably their only choice, was to draw the blood from Jeffrey's forehead.

After securing the oversized rubber band around his head, which they did with admirable gentleness, they attempted to draw blood. It failed. Jeffrey, wailing and producing tears again, turned gray, then white. I, too, felt void of any color, ready to pass out from the whole ordeal. That was no option, however, as he was the pin cushion, so I just cried again. Or more.

The nurses decided to try another spot on Jeffrey's forehead, and eventually, precious blood dripped into the tube. According to the specifications for the test, it wasn't quite enough, but the nurses opted to submit it to the lab, anyway. I'm sure there were prayers coming from their corner that the amount would be adequate. There were certainly plenty coming from mine.

It would take two weeks for us to get the results of the test… two weeks in which we could hope and pray that some sort of gross mistake had been made somewhere. Anywhere.

The next source of excruciating agony was the EMG (electromyelogram) to determine any muscle viability, or activity. It was considerably more miserable and longer in duration than either the x-ray or drawing of the blood for the genetic test.

In this test, an electrical current was zapped to various muscles in Jeffrey's legs to check for a response of any nature anywhere. As with the chest x-ray, Jeffrey and I both bawled throughout the entire procedure, his legs occasionally jerking from electrical connections as if he'd been struck by lightning.

I wasn't sure how there could be any tears left, as I felt quite certain I'd expelled a few decades' worth already. And how many more tricks could the medical monsters possibly have up their torturous white sleeves?

We must have reached our limit in God's eyes, as the worst of the medical ordeals ended with the EMG, at least for the time being. I was totally drained physically and emotionally, as was Jeffrey.

The procedures, necessary as they might have been, were grueling in every conceivable way, but it could have been worse. I could have been the one to make The Phone Call to my folks, Paul, and Nell, which Randy somehow managed.

I was certain I had had the easier deal.

Twenty

D r. Smith came in for another session, and my brain sparked long enough to ask some new questions:

Since Matthew and Katie hadn't shown symptoms yet, were they guaranteed safety from any type of SMA?

Should they be tested?

Was there a blood test to identify SMA before symptoms appeared?

For Jeffrey, what about cognitive abilities and language? Speech?

How fast was progression of the disease and regression of present abilities?

Just what does 'severe' mean?

Were there any restrictions?

Dr. Smith assured us a genetics counselor would be in to see us with answers to any questions we might have. While Dr. Usually Right exuded confidence in his assessments in general, he apparently didn't profess to know everything after all.

Before he escaped the threat of continued questions from Randy and me, I did manage to ask a final one: "What about the immunization shots?" His answer reeked of blunt insensitivity as he barely glanced up. "It doesn't really matter." The translation of that response, bolstered by his indifference, was clear, and I despised his nonchalance regarding the apparent premature death of our baby. Damn him.

The genetics counselor did materialize, and her compassion helped offset the concrete block personality of Dr. Smith. She said she had never heard of a family with different types of SMA, that it would be rare. It wasn't exactly the reassurance I wanted and needed in its entirety, but it would have to do. She tried to explain possible speech limitations and that usually cognitive abilities of those with SMA not only were not affected but, in fact, tended to be exceptional, regardless of the severity of physical limitations.

Her answers were vague. I knew why when she very carefully and quietly said, "And four is pretty old—most of the babies with Type 1 are gone by their second birthday."

Oh, God, no. More tears. Numb… and number. I could not imagine what it would take to sink into the numbest state available, but I had to be getting close.

On our second afternoon, the nurses (and Dr. Smith, who popped his smug, pessimistic head into the room) asked several times before dismissal if the social worker had come by yet. She hadn't. I felt sure we probably could have benefited from her visit, but we wanted to go home, to Matthew and Katie. Away from the insanity and hopelessness surrounding us.

Away from the promise of death.

Finally, at around 5:00 that afternoon, we asked if we could leave, despite the fact that the social worker had failed to appear. Sure, they said. Dr. Smith came into the room a final time and asked if we needed anything before we went home… other than a miracle, I supposed.

Thanks to my earlier experience teaching children with disabilities, I knew to ask if there was a support group for SMA, and he answered yes… and just stood there. Incredulous at his lack of interest in providing even a hint of assistance and support for us, I asked simply, "Um… could I have the number?"

His reaction indicated it was an inconvenience in his busy schedule of doling out devastation, but that was not my problem. He left the room and returned with the phone number of the group (Families of SMA), which I guarded with my life. That would be the first call I made in the morning, assuming I could feign adequate lucidity.

As if it were an afterthought, the doctor accompanying Dr. Smith asked me if Jeffrey had minded the EMG. Minded? I replied he had hated it and bawled the entire time. He replied with obvious surprise, "Really? Then there must be something there."

The screams of shock, disbelief, and utter fear permeated the confines of my head: *SOMETHING THERE? THEN DOES THAT MEAN THERE'S SOME HOPE? WHY DIDN'T YOU SAY SOMETHING EARLIER, JERK? WHAT IS GOING ON HERE? JEEPERS! DAMN YOU ALL!*

I wondered if these white coats had ever reflected not only on what they said—or didn't say—to families, but how they said it, if they had a clue as to how insensitive and arrogant their statements came off, how utterly helpless families felt in such dire circumstances, how willingly these 'pros' seemed to accept their roles as bearers of bad tidings. Probably not. Bedside manner was not something they were likely to learn from the pages of their textbooks. Or, apparently, cared to know.

I wondered if they'd ever know how lucky they were that *they* were not my priority.

Twenty-one

Upon our escape from the land of sterile white and stainless steel, wires, beeps, monitors, torture, and utter despair, we stopped at the office of a local chiropractor. Dr. Davidson* had been recommended to Randy by employees of a health food store in Winston during one of his searches to find something nutritious for us to eat.

The entire staff welcomed us as soon as we walked through the door. Dr. Davidson, putting us at ease immediately, expressed great interest in Jeffrey's case and wasted no time with his gentle examination. He found a spot on the side of Jeffrey's neck and began rubbing it, and in a matter of seconds, there was movement from Jeffrey's feet! He described the comparable location on a kitten's neck as the spot the mother cat licks to initiate movement by the newborn kitten.

We were instructed to massage that spot several times a day. Sheesh—I pledged to meow, grow fur, sprout whiskers and a tail, and give birth to kittens if it would help. It seemed easier than the alternative.

With heartfelt enthusiasm accompanying us, the ride home was much more animated than the ride from home had been just a day before. Randy and I began discussing the possibilities for our selection as Jeffrey's family and came up with one that sounded particularly reasonable to us. As we were interested in natural foods, maybe we would be the ones to discover a way to stop the muscle degeneration. Yes—that was it! That must be it!

For the first time in days, I was actually looking forward to something with my usual optimism rather than sheer dread, and that was a major accomplishment. We'd been handed a daunting assignment, and with my second wind, I now felt we were up to the task. With the help of the right folks and some hefty prayers, it wasn't unreasonable to think we might be able to unearth something that would keep Jeffrey with us, and, in the process, help others with SMA faced with the same devastation. How rejuvenated we felt!

About thirty miles from home, we had to stop at K-Mart for paper towels and dog food. How I managed to remember we needed them after the events of the past 72 hours was beyond my comprehension, but the mind, like the Lord, works in mysterious ways.

Everywhere I turned in the store, I was surrounded by baby and toddler things, and they all seemed to be boy items. I felt my soul breaking apart, one piece at a time. I shuffled from one aisle to another, numbly and stiffly, thanks to poison ivy, recent physical stagnation, sleep deprivation, and a wee bit of stress, searching for the two imperative items without dwelling on the surroundings taunting me.

The paper towels and dog food were located and purchased, and we continued up the mountain for home as our renewed optimism began drowning slowly in a flood of emotional, mental, and physical exhaustion.

We were almost home, though, where we all belonged. What we would say or do once we arrived and saw Matthew and Katie and my folks was anyone's guess. It called for another prayer request.

I'd be signing up for a lifetime membership on the prayer hotline to God.

Twenty-two

We had barely pulled into the driveway and opened the door when Mom and Dad arrived with Matthew and Katie. While it was a relief to have made it home and a blessing to be back with our family, I had to think particularly fast as to what I was about to say to any and all of them. Had I known then that my folks already knew plenty of details from Paul, I'm not sure if it would have been easier or tougher to report on our excursion with some semblance of optimism. Matthew and Katie settled themselves on the couch, ready to hear good news about their favorite baby brother.

I had just begun my attempt to relay positive aspects about the trip when I heard what sounded like digging somewhere outside. I looked out the window and saw Randy busy with a shovel, but I had no idea why he had to dig at that moment. Maybe he had flipped over into la-la land without me... just when I needed him beside me for moral support, if nothing else.

I sent Matthew outside to investigate, and when he returned, I asked him what was going on. He replied, "Something dug Duffy up. Dad's burying him again."

Heavens. Was there no end? Couldn't we even get through this critical discussion, or were we in such dire need for comic relief? *Was* that comic relief?

More likely, it was just the new status quo.

Whatever subsequently came out of my mouth, courtesy of the grace of God, I trusted made sufficient sense. I explained that we had a really big challenge ahead of us and that we were excited about the opportunity to tackle it. I fumbled around for more words that our lives would never be the same. Mom, who must also have been in her own state of shock, said later it was perfect, which, while I didn't believe it, was somewhat comforting, since I had had no authority over what words tumbled out of my mouth. That was probably a good thing.

It was difficult to tell just how much Matthew and Katie absorbed from the latest news bulletin and from the optimism I had attempted to muster with my brain fumes bordering on empty. It became painfully obvious at bedtime, though, when Matthew started asking detailed questions, all of which were leading up to the big one.

I very carefully explained to him that Jeffrey's muscles for moving, sucking, and swallowing would continue to deteriorate until the breathing muscles were also affected. No further explanation was required, as buckets of tears gushed out of Matthew's eyes. I was either too tired to join him at that time, or I felt I needed to be in charge. Or, more likely, maybe there just weren't any tears left in the holding tank.

That night, Jeffrey slept great and seemed even more beautiful than before. So peaceful. So innocent. So exquisite.

Like an angel.

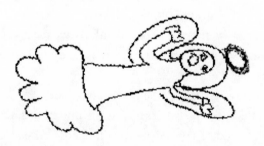

Twenty-three

After a fretful night of sleep, which would acquire a new, looser definition over the next few months, we faced the new day with a clear purpose, sense of direction, and an unexpectedly ample supply of adrenaline. Randy and Matthew left early for the far corners of the county and a few adjoining ones, searching for an alternative practitioner, or at least someone with expertise in the field of vitamins, minerals, and/or miracles. Meanwhile, Katie and I held down the fort with Jeffrey, getting our own ball rolling down other lanes.

My first order of business was to contact Families of SMA and request whatever information and support they could offer. It was surprisingly comforting to have on the other end of the line someone who knew all too well what I needed without my having to explain details, as I was not able to chat long without bursting into tears.

That accomplished, next came a call to renew my subscription to *Exceptional Parent* magazine, which had expired along with my teaching stint. Surely there was something in it that would help in some way.

Feeling quite confident about my success thus far, I welcomed the rain that began falling without warning in the middle of the sunshine. Fully expecting a good-news rainbow to materialize, I prepared for my next important phone call when a tremendous bolt of lightning zapped the phone line.

I couldn't use the bag car phone, as Randy and Matthew had taken it with them, nor, because of the lightning, could I send Katie to any of the neighbors' houses, all distant, to see if we all happened to be without phone service, or if it was just another test earmarked for us.

I didn't know what to do, except pray, now an automatic response. Not surprisingly, I was doing a lot of it… for Jeffrey, for my mental and emotional health, for the entire family, and now, for the phones. About that time, my folks made an angel appearance, arriving with a healthy lunch and returning to the lodge to call the phone company for me. The problem was a cable, and about 600 families were affected. Hallelujah—it wasn't just us after all! Mom and Dad brought their portable phone over, and I jumped back into business.

Needing to stretch my still-itching legs, I walked into the kitchen and spied huge black ants happily rummaging in the food on the dishes sitting idly on the counter. That was enough, but it wasn't as bad as the slug I spied on the kitchen floor… a really big slug. The final straw du jour. More tears.

I composed myself, then moved on to compose a 'Jeffrey letter,' begging mostly for prayers, but also for information regarding alternative therapy or even SMA. The first person on my list was Mary, the school nurse I had worked with at Brockman, based on my assumption that she might have access to the most potentially beneficial resources. The list went on from there to include those I had worked with in any capacity, former and current neighbors and friends, parents of Matthew and Katie's classmates (including those from preschool days). There were names of folks I knew would help if at all possible and those whose help I doubted, folks I liked, folks I didn't, and folks who probably wouldn't have a clue who I was. Pride was nonexistent; I would leave no stone unturned, no matter what might be underneath.

I just hoped there weren't too many slugs.

Twenty-four

Randy and Matthew returned home late after a profitable day of abundant discoveries, beginning with the fact that the car had been on the verge of losing all its wheels and the realization of the miracle that they hadn't come off on our way to or from Winston-Salem.

Randy also reported that they had unearthed an alternative practitioner who knew Dr. Smith (I hoped they weren't peas from the same pod) and who had shared some hopeful information about different natural supplements. Randy had bought some of the recommended supplements to get Jeffrey started until we were able to get him in for an appointment.

All in all, it was a good, productive day for both teams with some significant accomplishments. One of the biggest, I thought, was that I hadn't been locked up in a rubber room.

The next morning, I squirted one of the new Evening Primrose capsules into Jeffrey's mouth, his expression indicating he thought the whole thing was pretty silly. I felt a sense of success and decided that he would make this ordeal much easier than I'd dreamed possible.

I then readied twenty Jeffrey letters to mail out, including a request to be placed on the *Guideposts* prayer list. Dad brought a loaf of bread over, and a home health nurse popped in unannounced. She'd tried to provide notice of her visit, but the phones were still out. She was kind in her exam and questioning and attempted to answer a question I'd silently practiced asking—whether or not Jeffrey's organs could be donated when it was 'time.' She said she thought an individual had to be hooked up to life support in order for the organs to remain viable for transplant, but she'd check.

As she spoke, I watched an ant crawl over the back of her chair while an earwig escaped from under one of the many pairs of shoes strewn on the floor. I hoped she wouldn't need to go to the bathroom, as the daddy long legs had taken up residence there, even on the toilet paper. It was anyone's guess as to what might escape from the enormous pile of clothes on the couch; I prayed it would be nothing boasting hair and a tail.

After the nurse left, I pumped some breast milk for Jeffrey so I could add the new batch of supplements. By the time I finished preparing the concoction and handed the bottle of gold to Matthew to give Jeffrey, our little fellow was sound asleep.

At the end of the first day of steady prayers and supplements, there was a change in Jeffrey—a slightly tighter hand grip, movement of his forearm several times, louder cry, slight plantar reflex movement in both feet, and a bit of head control for a few seconds longer than ever while I held him in a sitting position. Maybe that was what we had been learning—the power of faith and prayer. And we must have been fast learners. It was a miracle!

Thank you, dear Lord!

Twenty-five

July 18—Matthew's eleventh birthday! I stuck eleven dollars in an envelope as a mini-celebratory gesture, and he replied, "Wow—I can't wait until I'm fifty!" My gift to me, besides the memories of Matthew's birth and the past eleven speedy years, was a sweet dream the night before that Jeffrey was able to bear weight on his legs.

Mom brought over a huge Lego set for Matthew and a few new Beanie Babies for Katie. Jeffrey's gift arrived from a medical supply company in the form of a suction machine for *just in case*. The delivery man, through no fault of his own, didn't realize his arrival was a bummer and simply asked if I knew how to work the piece of equipment, as he wasn't sure. I assured him I did because I'd used the same kind on my trached student at Brockman; I was just hoping I wasn't going to have to use it, at least any time soon. I knew the necessity of the suction machine would signal the end of Jeffrey's ability to swallow.

To celebrate Matthew's big day, made even more joyous when Jeffrey lifted both forearms instead of sliding them up on his lap pillow, Dad took Matthew and Katie to dinner and a movie—no doubt, the best thing that had happened to them in some time. They even issued a self-imposed cease-fire from their normal verbal battles for a few hours.

While they were gone, I read information Paul had mailed about SMA, particularly that it generally claimed total victory (i.e., death) anywhere from a few months to three years in its Type 1 destruction mode. It wasn't enjoyable reading, but I craved information, truly believing that while our faith in God was our armor, information about SMA was our weapon (I must have read that somewhere; my brain was totally incapable of original profound philosophical pronouncements). We would need an ample supply of both faith and information.

The next evening, I received a phone call from the first batch of Jeffrey letters! A friend provided the name of a doctor who treated patients with a combination of traditional and nontraditional therapy, certainly worthy of further inquiry after the weekend. Two more calls came, both from former teaching buddies with helpful suggestions. I was eager for the phone to ring and to hear other avenues we might be able to consider on our quest to end this cruel joke.

While I thought Randy and I were holding up remarkably well, relatively speaking, I was concerned about Matthew and Katie. They seemed to be fine, although I knew they had to be experiencing significant inner turmoil. I tried to discuss stress with them and the need for each of us to release 'stress poisons' in our own way and time. In a nutshell, we would fall apart individually, in small groups, or simultaneously for an unknown duration of time. We would be an exceptionally merry bunch for a while, but maybe we'd be able to retain a smidgen of sanity in this lunacy. Maybe.

Randy, out on errands, called to report that he had locked the keys in the car, which was still running. Of course, the air conditioning was on to cool the organic eggs that needed to be refrigerated ASAP unless we wanted baby chickens on the loose. Not really. Murphy's Law prevailed, even in the face of tragedy.

Well, we *were* trying to keep things as normal as possible.

Twenty-six

Randy, Jeffrey, and I made our initial trip to Dr. Cade*, the chiropractor/alternative practitioner, on July 21, one week after the diagnosis. It was a surprisingly upbeat visit, as Dr. Cade, who had been reading about SMA, was pleased to see what Jeffrey could do.

After taking a history from us and examining his tiny new patient, he gave us the names of a few supplemental minerals, vitamins, and herbs on top of what Randy had already purchased, along with some exercises to do with Jeffrey.

The subsequent schedule would depend on Jeffrey and what improvement, if any, was noticed. Dr. Cade explained that any regimen designed for Jeffrey would be purely experimental, based on known benefits of individual components. We understood that we had nothing to lose and possibly everything to gain, should it work to any degree. We left the office in good spirits and with a few scheduled appointments for the following week.

Our lingering optimism from Dr. Cade came to a screeching halt in late afternoon, when Matthew began complaining of mild pain in his right side. When the pain worsened as the evening progressed, the only course of action was for Randy to take him to the emergency room. I needed to stay with Jeffrey; we had no pumped milk for emergencies, and I didn't want to lug him to the hospital, not knowing what developments or germs were lurking.

Expectations of the phone's ringing with news of a ruptured appendix and emergency surgery jump-started my imagination, and my head began pounding with the thought that I had let Matthew down for not being there with him. I had managed to play nursemaid to him and Katie whenever they were sick and hated that I had had to make a choice, even though there really was no choice.

I knew in my brain that Randy was perfectly competent, yet I tried in vain to figure out how I could be there and with Jeffrey, too. Katie was fast asleep, and I knew Mom or Dad or both would be right over if necessary, but the logistics simply wouldn't jibe. No solution. More prayers. More dreading the phone to ring.

It was the beginning of a necessary revelation that I simply couldn't do it all myself.

Miraculously, the phone didn't ring; instead, Randy and Matthew returned home. Apparently, there was an elevation of something noted in an allergy test the doctor had run. Allergy!

Matthew would be fine… unless he had an allergy to stress.

Twenty-seven

The days turned almost cheery again, thanks to the support and prayers pouring in, some from friends, former colleagues, and neighbors, but mostly from folks we would never meet. I became more aware of an intense connection to God, a connection I knew had to remain steadfast if I expected to get through this and share any optimistic vibes with the rest of the family. Already my prayers to God, sincere in the purest sense, had shifted from those of desperation and negotiation immediately following the diagnosis (*Please, PLEASE, I'll do anything, just please don't take Jeffrey. PLEASE.*) to requests for the courage, wisdom, and strength to handle this assignment. I also prayed, strangely enough, for the ability to find humor. Anywhere.

One morning, Katie and I ran several errands, all in the name of Jeffrey, including picking up more Jeffrey letters at the printer's and delivering a few of them wherever we stopped around town. At Social Services, where we picked up gas vouchers for the medical appointments, one of the counselors looked at my leg, still plagued madly with poison ivy, and asked, "What did you do to your leg?" As we left, Katie remarked, "I thought she was talking about my leg, 'cause it's so hairy."

What an incredible gift Katie possessed, whether she realized it or not—the ability to retain her wits and humor during adversity and make a difference for someone else. She had inadvertently just served as an answer to one of my prayers!

Thank heavens for children… and hairy legs.

Twenty-eight

July 24 was a big day in several ways. Matthew and Katie worked with Randy in his fledgling carpet dry-cleaning business, earning money for their efforts. Matthew had already spied a gigantic Lego set on which to spend his earnings, while Katie spent at least as much effort mastering the time-clock as she did working. Jeffrey was placed on the prayer list of 100,000 Goldwingers, a group of motorcycle riders, some of whom had stayed at the lodge in the past.

Someone was to come the following day to set us up with the Internet. It was certain to tax my insufficient gray matter, as I had never laid eyes on the Internet, but it would provide a vital link to information regarding SMA and medical advancements. Perhaps an even more essential component of this technical wonder would be the ability to connect with other SMA families. I had to have it and without delay.

I loaded Jeffrey in the carseat for our first solo appointment with Dr. Cade and started crying as soon as I reached the end of our driveway… our very short driveway. I must have been in serious need of stress reduction, as I bawled the entire distance of about thirty-five miles. Apparently, I wasn't yet fully acclimated to the emotional turbulence of our recent days, and it was as obvious as the tenacious poison ivy on my legs.

I somehow regained enough composure to locate the office, but I almost lost it again when Dr. Cade tended to us hurriedly. He gave Jeffrey a quick spinal and cranial adjustment and said he'd see him the following week to check for any signs of improvement. Then, either forgetting our other appointments previously scheduled or no longer seeing the need for them, he explained that we'd set up a tentative schedule, communicating via e-mail, which we didn't even have yet. End of visit.

Next, please...

After the appointment, which had failed to provide the anticipated boost to my spirits, Jeffrey and I made a few stops, leaving Jeffrey letters at each of them. We arrived home to numerous phone calls from friends rallying with potentially useful information, as well as a visit from Matthew's fifth-grade teacher, with whom I'd volunteered regularly the previous year. She had heard about Jeffrey from her husband, who worked at the phone company and learned I had inquired about placement on an emergency list. Before leaving, she quietly slipped an envelope into my hand; it contained an incredibly generous donation to the Jeffrey cause. That same afternoon, her husband called from the phone company to let us know we would receive courtesy Internet service for at least six months. The earth angels kept coming, and we needed and appreciated them all.

Dad stopped by a church in town during the afternoon, apparently feeling the need for divine inspiration and/or reassurance. He mentioned Jeffrey to the minister, who told him he had already heard about Jeffrey—his wife was the one coming to set us up on the Internet the next day! Coincidence? No. I had already been convinced that there were no coincidences, just connecting pieces of God's puzzle of Life.

More prayers... this time, of thanks to God for providing so many beams of hope to hold us together and upright.

God is great, God is good...

Twenty-nine

om's paternal first cousin in California has two grand-daughters with what I'd somehow understood through the years was spina bifida; having never met them, I had no reason to question my assumption. Mom received a letter from her cousin, in which she mentioned the girls' muscle disease. Knowing that spina bifida was not a muscle disease, I asked Mom to find out (rather, confirm) what they had.

Mom called later in the day to report she had learned the answer from her sister, Peggy, who had written down the information years ago and, amazingly, knew exactly where to find it. SMA. The girls were diagnosed at a later age than Jeffrey and, consequently, have a milder type, but still... Now successful young women, both were leaders in school, bright, outgoing, industrious, happy, pretty, and popular with their classmates. They provided a unique family link and history for Jeffrey, and I planned to find some time to communicate with them.

The rest of the day was packed, as they all seemed to be, but as long as there was even a hint of positive direction, I didn't dare complain. One of the items involved the addition of a second brain to the treatment team.

Dr. Hendrix* was another chiropractor I'd heard was specially trained in cranial adjustments, a lost-art technique supposedly vital for optimal health. Whereas Dr. Cade reminded me of Richard Dreyfuss, coming off as somewhat brusque and cocky more often than not (though not nearly as proficient at it as our favorite neurologist), Dr. Hendrix reminded me of Bill Cosby, upbeat and relaxed, his calming vibes providing a welcomed balance to Dr. Cade's somewhat arrogant manner. It was almost like having a taste of show business.

And together, we'd try to keep this show afloat as long as possible.

Thirty

D
r. Hendrix was fascinated with Jeffrey on the initial visit and eager to discover what might be done. Jeffrey's smile performed its magic on all who were around, including a mother whose child had been in a recent swimming class with Matthew and Katie. She sold vitamins and reported that Dr. Hendrix was her husband's cousin. She said she would spread copies of the Jeffrey letter around, even to the local radio station.

Now we were getting somewhere.

After the first appointment with Dr. Hendrix, Jeffrey and I then headed to Dr. Cade, who was much more patient than he had been on the previous visit and actually demonstrated his adequate baby-chatting skills with Jeffrey. I was again confident with our decision to use him as our primary doctor, with Dr. Hendrix as the secondary pro. I planned to keep looking around, though, just in case there might be a medicine man to toss into the pot. I would consider snake oil, witch doctors, and magic wands.

We returned home in relatively fine form, and I received an exciting phone call. A friend said an acquaintance was scheduled to attend a convention the following month with 2,000 alternative practitioners, and she was planning to share Jeffrey's story! We had a mini-celebrity around, yet there was no glory going to his head. Too bad it wasn't going to his muscles, either. Yet.

Murphy's Law continued with the Internet hookup, but after hours of work spanning two days and a replacement for the defective first modem, we were finally set up.

Instantly, our world expanded in ways I could never have imagined. I was directed right away by the computer gal to the web site for Families of SMA, where I found a message posted on our behalf from a friend in South Carolina! Incredible.

When our computer gal left, I got online to experiment, then Randy got on, then Matthew, then Katie, then I got on again (well, someone had to use Jeffrey's turn). We already needed four computers and four Internet lines!

And many, many more prayers.

Thirty-one

My days were fully occupied with Jeffrey duties: massaging his arms and legs and trunk and neck and fingers and toes, mixing the miracle concoctions, pumping milk, nursing, changing diapers, exercising his legs, more massaging, nursing, infant stimulation activities, cuddling, nursing, rocking, etc., etc., etc. There was also the answering of Matthew's questions, management of Katie's emotional explosions, and refereeing of spats between the two of them, but I somehow grabbed time to search the Internet for medical information as well as other families tossed into the same black hole.

It was absolutely indescribable to feel so connected to the rest of the world even in our midst of cow pastures and wild turkeys. What a surge of optimism I felt in clicking my way down paths that sometimes led to what were surely secret chambers in the world of medical wonder.

I was completely enthralled with my newfound ability to discover all there was to know about SMA (not much), although I understood only a portion of what I read. The amount of material I unearthed seemed rather scant but was enough to keep me searching for more information and any amount of hope.

Even better, being able to communicate with other SMA families via the magic of the Internet provided immense mental and emotional fortification. Social communication over and above waving at carpool or cheering together at ball games was tough in this rural area. With the Internet, however, I was communicating with families across the world, and as we shared plights, we understood each other well.

A bonus of online communication was that I could sob the

entire time while typing a message and yet could possibly still be perceived as relatively coherent... most of the time, anyway. I could not comprehend how folks dealt with SMA (or any other devastating situation) without Internet access to other SMA families and the cyber hugs they sent out to each other so readily... and that we all snatched up with gratitude.

What I didn't fully realize then was the inner strength I was harvesting by reading messages from families who had already lost a baby... or worse, more than one. Their ability to form complete sentences and express positive thoughts was, unbeknownst to me at the time, invigorating my subconscious for the future.

I kept telling myself we would get through this and be stronger, thanks to the vital acquisition of information and family contacts. And prayer.

Plenty of times I wondered, though, just what price we'd pay for our character building.

Thirty-two

In order to inform ourselves and the doctors, who also knew virtually nothing about SMA, I continued reading as much as possible. Countering the sobering facts and similar stories of Type 1 babies with enough optimism to absorb it all without wallowing in depression was not easy.

The diagnosis is typically made before three months; physical milestones are never accomplished; swallowing and feeding are difficult, and the respiratory muscles are weak; respiratory infections are usually frequent and serious; prognosis is poor; death in the majority of children usually occurs by the age of two. No treatment or cure.

Meanwhile, the days zoomed by. No matter how hard I tried or how fast I worked, I never managed to finish what I thought was important, and that did not include housecleaning. To complicate life, my fuzzy brain couldn't distinguish between 'SMA' events and 'normal baby' ones, such as Jeffrey's increased drooling. Was it from weakened swallowing muscles or teething? I began feeling incompetent as both a mother and nurse.

Matthew and Katie managed to demonstrate an impressive general resilience to the adversity, mostly with the humor I craved. Katie's occasional song outburst was occasionally enhanced by a banana microphone, and Matthew exclaimed, after witnessing a substantial expulsion of gas from Jeffrey, "Wow—I hope that isn't the highlight of my day!" It was a welcomed relief from the tension that continued mounting, testing my sanity and stripping my nerves, which already felt completely naked.

One of the countless final straws snapped when I spent a

valuable hour preparing a report of Jeffrey's treatment for a nutritionist who had requested it. I gathered all the supplement bottles from the kitchen and carted them to the computer desk, carefully charting the names, dosages, and other details of the lengthy treatment regimen. I clicked *Print* on the computer and returned the armload of bottles to the kitchen.

When I returned to what should have been a printout of my laborious efforts, nothing was waiting for me. Absolutely nothing had happened in my absence... and then I realized the computer had frozen and that I would have to repeat the entire process because, of course, I hadn't thought to save it first. In a flood of tears, I trudged back to the kitchen, gathered the bottles once again, and trudged back to the computer. The sobbing was uncontrollable by that time, no doubt due to the now-standard lack of sleep and the fact that I had been reading the consistently dismal outlook for Type 1 babies for too long. A dark rubber room sounded increasingly attractive.

As I was pondering what one packed for the rubber room, a good friend called to relay what she had just heard on the radio—*God gives us what we need when we need it.* She had felt compelled to share it with us right then.

Once again, He had sent an earth angel... when I needed one... just as the letter I'd been dreading arrived in the mail, wiping out all hopes for an error in lab work, an error in Dr. Usually Right's confident, smug diagnosis, an error in prognosis, an error in placement of our family in this hell of a nightmare.

SMA, confirmed.

Thirty-three

On the third day of August, we managed to throw together Matthew's belated birthday party at the park down the road. Hot dogs, cake, friends, presents, baseball, and laughter resulted in a welcomed touch of everyone else's real world.

Four days later, school began for Matthew (sixth grade) and Katie (third grade). After sparse joys of the summer, both were eager to return to the routine school would provide. A routine of normalcy. Of safety. Both raved about their new teachers, who would likely have greater issues with them than reading, writing, math, and homework. I trusted we'd all be ready.

On the 11th, Randy and I took Jeffrey back to Dr. Smith in Winston-Salem for the previously scheduled neurological re-check, eager to hear what Dr. Doom would have to say about the slight increase in movement Jeffrey now demonstrated in his arms and legs.

When Dr. Smith stepped into the office, he seemed surprised to see us at all, but I attributed it to my anticipation of a pessimistic reaction from him and ignored it. He examined Jeffrey, who moved as if on cue, and said nothing while jotting notes, even though he seemed mildly curious about the increased movement. He did mumble some guarded comment about a so-called medical basis for the increased movement, declining to elaborate on a level a human could understand, and that was it.

I couldn't contain myself any longer. I rattled off our strict adherence to the custom-designed treatment regimen of vitamins, herbs, minerals, physical stimulation, and prayer, and our noticing an almost immediate increase of movement. Dr. Smith scribbled a few additional notes without any acknowledgment that we were in the room. He told us to check into an experimental program in Dallas, Texas, set for October, which would test a drug on SMA babies that is normally reserved for patients with ALS (amyotrophic lateral sclerosis, or Lou Gehrig's disease), considered by some to be a variation of SMA. He then instructed us to bring Jeffrey back in a few months. End of exam, end of discussion.

Before Randy and I left his office in disbelief over his lack of even pretend interest in Jeffrey or in us, we decided we wouldn't drag Jeffrey there again; this medical 'expert' apparently couldn't—or wouldn't—provide much in the way of encouragement, and we had long since surpassed our quota of discouragement.

We then headed to the office of Dr. Davidson, the chiropractor, for a replenishment of optimism. He expressed genuine delight at Jeffrey's progress and called in his staff, all hovering on the opposite side of the door in anticipation of a formal invitation inside the room. Dr. Davidson and his caring staff more than compensated for Dr. Doom's lack of encouragement. They would remain with us on our journey.

We celebrated the good vibes by heading over to Sagebrush for lunch, tossing peanut shells onto the floor until it reminded us of home. Not that we toss peanut shells on the floor at home for character. Don't need to.

The improvement in Jeffrey's movement and cry, becoming delightfully loud, and even the barest hint of a reflex impacted us all, but it especially boosted the morale of Matthew and Katie. Every day after school, Matthew asked eagerly if Jeffrey had had a good day. I wanted to be honest in a positive way, and I reported every detail that seemed even remotely optimistic. "Yes! he stayed awake longer today!," or "Yes! he moved his legs more!," or "Yes! he smiled whenever he was awake!"

Katie bypassed what she considered frivolous inquiries and rushed over to Jeffrey as soon as she bolted through the door each afternoon, cooing to him boisterously and jerking his legs back and forth until I thought they would disengage in self-defense. Any time I reminded her to be careful, however, Jeffrey beamed with even more adoration at his favorite big sister.

With the exception of this initial Jeffrey jostle each day, though, Katie became increasingly irritable, a justifiable side effect from a level of stress even adults grappled with uneasily. Thankfully, it didn't extend to school.

We had more talks on Jeffrey's probable future and God's reason for it all, including His decision to place us all together as a family in the first place. Despite a wide variety of possible explanations, though, all we knew for sure was that we had no real clue about anything… and probably shouldn't count on getting the answers any time soon, either. Considering our lack of insider information, we just had to believe (and did) that God had a particularly good reason for handing us this assignment.

If our faith in the goodness of God ever faltered, we were sunk.

Thirty-four

August 19—Katie's eighth birthday! She packed her eight birthday dollars for the book fair at school, claiming she loved to read. She did (used to) love to read, but I knew she mainly loved to spend money.

After she and Matthew left for school, I noticed Jeffrey's nursing was slurpy, and I tried to formulate possible theories in an effort to skirt the most obvious reason. I felt jittery all day, probably also in part because Jeffrey slept through most of it; however, as he managed to take his fist to his mouth and suck it, that served as a Happy Katie's Birthday present to us all!

That afternoon, unusually hot, I gathered baby stuff, Jeffrey, and a generous supply of popsicles to take to Katie and her classmates at school before the final bell rang. All was fine until I tried to park in the parking lot. I found an empty spot fairly close to her class on the playground and had just finished unloading everything, including Jeffrey, in the broiling sun as a man sauntered up and said, "You're in a bus driver's spot, and that driver won't be too happy if his space is taken."

I likely could have flooded the parking lot with the tears that had been gathering momentum for a prime moment in which to burst forth. I considered this a prime-enough moment but held back as best I could. Tears were hardly on the agenda for a popsicle birthday bash.

Without a word or gesture (of any nature), I quietly bit my lip, took a deep breath, buckled Jeffrey back into his seat, shoved everything back into the car, and drove around until I thought I had found a safe spot, if there was such a thing in the parking lot. Or in life itself, for that matter.

The mini-party went fine, and Katie's mood was festive until Matthew got into the car after school and reached for a leftover popsicle. Whoa. So much for the birthday girl's gracious hostess skills and party disposition…

The next steamy day was another two-doctor adventure. Despite our running late and Jeffrey's indignation at having to demonstrate his sucking reflexes on a rubber glove (yum), the day was almost easy until we tried to leave the parking lot at Wal-Mart, which had become a routine post-appointment excursion. The car refused to start. I called Randy, who reminded me there was an automotive department right there, then lugged Jeffrey back into the store and seventeen miles back to the automotive department.

I explained what had happened and was told to wait, that someone would be with me as soon as possible. Right. Confident I was stuck for a while in the stale nook because that's the way it always is, I unstrapped Jeffrey and got him ready for a bottle I'd brought and needed to use. My reaching for the bottle promptly signaled the contents of Jeffrey's bag to spill out all over the basket and down to the floor.

As soon as everything was sufficiently scattered under the gumball machines and over every other square inch of grungy linoleum, I heard, "He's ready, Ma'am." But of course. Not knowing when my next bit of assistance would materialize if I didn't accept, and seeing that Jeffrey was just as happy dozing, I put the sleepy guy back into his carseat, gathered up what I could see on the cootie-laden floor, and pushed the basket back to the scorching parking lot.

The battery was too dead to register on the charger, so Jeffrey and I had the pleasure of trudging into the store once again to purchase a replacement, uttering thanks that if the battery had to die, at least it happened at a store with an on-site automotive department.

With our new battery installed, I proceeded to provide it with significant initiation into our routine of chaos. I rushed home, gulping a Big Mac on the way, fed and changed Jeffrey and put drops in his eye for a goopy eye infection he'd recently developed, flew to a screening meeting for PACT (Parents and Children Together) to see what services might be available for Jeffrey, then zipped back across the county afterwards to the lodge to pick up Matthew and Katie.

We headed back home for spelling, writing, health, reading, and whatever else was on the homework agenda, while Randy scrounged up something for dinner, a chore he'd accepted without hesitation or complaint. I tried connecting to the Internet for an information search, but the line stayed busy. I could relate.

The day closed with a slug sighting... on the kitchen table.

Thirty-five

The month of August was almost history. It had been relatively uneventful in the catastrophe department but plenty full of teasers. I noticed a slightly crusty orange stain in Jeffrey's diaper, which I attributed to his vitamins. I refused to panic because he didn't act like he felt bad; however, I did contact Paul, who, based on my description of something orange and crusty in Jeffrey's diaper, had no idea what it could be. Matthew had used his inhaler a few days *just in case*, he said. It was a miracle we were not all on inhalers... or worse.

We survived Katie's birthday party at the lodge, with a beautiful cake provided by an earth angel mom who had insisted on bringing one. Our Jeffrey journey had certainly relaxed my need to be completely self-sufficient. I would never have even pondered tossing cake duty for my own child to someone else in the past. SMA had reduced my ability to perform even the simplest, normal mommy duties to the absolute minimum... as if what I was doing for Jeffrey was simple or minimal. Or normal.

I found an exciting entry in the Families of SMA (FSMA) Guest Book that evening. A mom from North Carolina, whose young son had Type 2, had recently returned from the national FSMA conference with her family, rejuvenated and resolved to start an FSMA chapter in our state! I eagerly began answering her note, expressing genuine interest in helping however I could, when I was suddenly interrupted by a big thud outside, right where the corner column of the house was.

Rather, right where it used to be.

Luckily, Randy had supported the corner with a two-by-four a few months earlier so we wouldn't collapse when the post rotted away. We hadn't bothered to remove the post because of the bluebird family that had taken up residence; we had been reminded all too recently that we were at the beck of Mother Nature's calls, and not vice versa.

Somehow *we* hadn't collapsed (yet), but we were apparently getting closer in more ways than one. I tried not to view the post's fall as an omen and looked forward to helping out with the proposed local chapter of support, 'local' as in three hours across the state.

I didn't realize then that I was reaping another blessing courtesy, ironically, of SMA. The mom, Cindy Schaefer, would soon become one of my closest fellow warriors in the SMA battle we both fought, and our friendship would soon transcend the boundaries of the challenge that brought us together.

I began needing to suction Jeffrey's nose with the bulb syringe frequently, attributing it to the allergy season that had included most of the family in its wrath, and, at the suggestion of the doctor, used a saline solution to help with his congestion.

Immediately after the drops were placed in Jeffrey's nose, he sputtered, reddened, and gasped for breath, leading me to believe that not only was it the beginning of the end, but that it wouldn't be pleasant. The prayers, like the mama issuing them, were frantic. He recovered his spunk quickly enough, while I was left trembling and relieved that I was already collapsed in the chair.

I realized then that almost every bit of disruption could be attributed to SMA and its propensity for catastrophe. Even though many of the occurrences also affected normal, healthy children, there would be no releasing of the guard here. Simple, seemingly innocuous colds and upper respiratory infections had hair-raising potential to send babies, children, and adults with SMA into ICU for extensive stays; some never made it back home. With

Jeffrey cast into a precarious position in the deadliest form of the killer disease, there would be no casual reaction to anything respiratory. From now on, sneezes, coughs, and a stuffy nose would sound the alarm, necessarily or not. I felt sure I wouldn't be able to discern between a crisis-in-the-making or simply self-defense in response to the dust farm in the house. How long could I possibly hold up with my self-confidence as a mama and nurse in shambles? More prayers.

The last day of the month was marked with news of Princess Diana's death in a car crash. As shocking and tragic as it was, her death seemed almost fitting in our personal world now.

That seemed like the real tragedy.

Thirty-six

With August out of the way, surely September would be better. Or possibly worse, which was hardly any consolation. At any rate, it had one less day in it for disaster, and I considered that with great favor.

I took Jeffrey to a Brain Gym session, which would supposedly assist me in terms of dealing with stress and Jeffrey in terms of who-knew-what. It was certainly an interesting experience. The gal conducting it had a baby boy about a month older than Jeffrey, and we compared as many notes as we dared up to the obvious distinction.

My pint-sized charge fussed much of the time while I was being 'de-stressed,' rendering the session more than a little counterproductive. A few tears escaped there, and the rest fell out all the way home. I wondered if my stress level would ever drop to acceptable levels again, with or without help.

Mother Teresa died on the fifth day of the month. After Princess Diana's premature death only days before, I did not consider that a good sign at all, regardless of the fact that Mother Teresa was not exactly in the prime of youth. I briefly pondered the *bad luck runs in threes* superstition and was thankful I wasn't superstitious. Or hadn't been.

One day early in the month, Jeffrey napped in his crib instead of my lap, and I heard a strange noise escaping on the monitor. I rushed upstairs to see what excitement was brewing, incredulous to discover that what I had heard was nothing more than a cow across the road attempting to stir up some bovine conversation.

It's a pretty sad state when a mother confuses her child with a member of another species. I had no doubt that I would be carted away any day by unanimous decision.

I needed to start packing.

Thirty-seven

September 10 was dreadful. On our way down the mountain to the two doctors' visits, a sound completely unidentifiable other than a massive burp-cough came out of Jeffrey, and it scared off the remaining few wits I could claim. He seemed fine afterwards, but I battled heart palpitations the rest of the lengthy trip.

After two uneventful exams and the usual chiropractic adjustments, we dared to alter our usual post-doctor route to include K-Mart instead of Wal-Mart; it was about the only variation in our routine I felt capable of handling.

After only a few minutes in the store, I looked into the shopping basket to check my passenger, observing with great alarm Jeffrey's opening his mouth as if to whine, with nothing coming out. Like a fish out of water gasping for breath, his mouth didn't utter a peep. There was, however, no mistaking the terror in his eyes. And in mine.

I located a nearby dressing room with a bench within seconds and immediately whisked him out of his seat, hoping to elicit noise of any sort out of him. Nothing. I patted him on the back and tried to nurse him. Nothing. Headed towards a panic state and continuing to poke, pat, pound, prod, and pray, I wondered how loudly I could yell for help, fearing my efforts would resemble Jeffrey's, the screams imprisoned in my own head and heart. His diaper was soaked to the brim, so while frantically trying to conjure up some tricks, I dug a new diaper out for a quick change, praying feverishly that something intelligent would come to me soon. As if a switch had been flipped, Jeffrey's open mouth began uttering sounds as soon as the diaper was changed!

Tears flowed in profuse supply, as did the prayers of thanks, and we aborted our K-Mart expedition as soon as I thought I could stand and wobble to the car and then drive thirty miles back up the mountain. I wanted to go home, which I felt was fast becoming the only place that possessed any semblance of a safety net.

And only God knew when we would lose that.

Thirty-eight

Jeffrey's noisy gurgles on September 13 warranted my breaking out the suction machine. I managed to get him situated for his first suctioning experience without a total emotional breakdown, an accomplishment in itself, and flipped the switch to *ON*.

It sounded like it had marbles in it (I'd wondered where mine had gone), so I made a phone call to the medical equipment company for a replacement. I finally convinced the person on the other end that I did know what I was talking about by turning the machine on and holding the receiver up to the loudest spot. With ears no doubt ringing like a beginners' bell choir, the representative promised a replacement would be delivered soon.

A part of me was sorry the machine didn't work, but a larger part was relieved, as no one had asked me if I was ready for this chapter. I wasn't. I knew we would need to suction when Jeffrey's swallowing muscles were unable to handle his saliva, and that day would come soon enough. Perhaps it already had.

In lieu of modern technology, I turned on the hot shower for a couple of steam baths during the day and increased the chest PT, and it seemed to work in easing Jeffrey's gurgling. After we returned home from afternoon carpool, the new machine arrived. I was thankful for the speedy service, while secretly hoping it would not have to be dragged into action any time soon. Dreamer.

After more than enough serious bickering between Matthew and Katie later that afternoon, I asked them to list their priorities, thinking it was again time for us to regroup and discover things for which we could be thankful. Matthew's priorities were family, God, and Jeffrey. Katie listed hers as Jeffrey, family, Nellie,

God, and Wishbone, PBS' Jack Russell wonder canine. Spontaneous, unprofessional therapy accomplished a brief respite from the quarreling, for which my head was most appreciative.

On September 14, I determined that while we weren't facing a dire emergency yet, an opportunity for serious suctioning had arrived in earnest. I set the machine up on the kitchen table, placed Jeffrey in a 'working' position, turned the machine on, and bawled throughout the procedure, feeling that without question, this signaled a key element of the downslide. His ability to swallow was diminishing.

Our little fellow tolerated the procedure with ease, and I thanked God for affording me the opportunity to practice suctioning on my trached student, Tina, during my last year at Brockman. When I realized Jeffrey needed a second suctioning later in the day, I shifted to nurse mode and proceeded not with tears as much as a vague sense of depression justifiably attributed to fatigue, full moon, premonition, pessimism, and/or realism... or probably all of them knotted together in a single mind-boggling wad.

The bright spot, as usual, was Jeffrey's dazzling smile, letting me know he felt just great, thanks to the suctioning and all the TLC lavished on him, and daring to defy the cruel progression of SMA. I could tell the machine would be a mixed blessing, and I knew I should be thankful however our blessings arrived.

Randy commented later in the day that the house was a wreck (*Gee, Honey, I hadn't noticed*) and that someone would surely drop by. I confidently assured him it wasn't messy enough yet for visitors. I was wrong. A knock on the door revealed none other than the minister from the little church down the road. Randy reluctantly invited our brave visitor inside to Tornado Alley, where he eventually unearthed a spot on the couch, completely buried in towels, socks, and, of course, underwear.

At least they were clean.

Thirty-nine

According to so-called experts, the use of therapeutic electrical stimulation (TES) to stimulate muscle response was not indicated in patients with SMA. I figured those 'experts' did not also happen to be the parents of someone with SMA who had a guaranteed early date with death, so I was thrilled when Dr. Cade agreed to try it with Jeffrey.

With increased suctioning coming into the picture, and contact with families who had already lost their babies on the upswing, I felt the urgency of the situation mounting daily. I did not ever want to grapple with guilt that we could have tried something but didn't... because *they* said it wouldn't help.

Who were *they*, anyway, and what did they know? Probably not what I knew. Options for babies with Type 1 were virtually nil, with the exception of suctioning and chest PT to make them somewhat more comfortable for a bit longer. I knew this trial of TES was very possibly the end of the line of hope for Jeffrey, although we would continue it only if we felt confident that his quality of life was not being compromised.

Meanwhile, Randy and I attempted to keep life normal in as many aspects as possible. What a joke. Randy cooked, cleaned, ran errands, and took care of Matthew and Katie, all while trying to establish his carpet dry-cleaning business, still in its infancy. I primarily tended to Jeffrey as both mother and nurse, noticing everything about him and his ways and trying to decipher the changes as rationally as possible. If he nursed less, I wondered if it was a deterioration of the sucking muscles. If he slept more, was it because of SMA's excessive energy demands just for breathing?

It was a 24-hour alert-watch every day, and while my body was pushed above and beyond, it was performing without a sputter. It became apparent just how incredibly effectively we can function when there is no other choice. And if we pray a lot.

While I was pulling mama/nurse duty, Randy was having his own Jeffrey moments at times. While cleaning the carpet at Badger Funeral Home, he bumped into a small box… with an infant casket inside. He somehow managed to regroup and forged ahead, knowing that this was where Jeffrey's service would be. Would that be *our* baby's casket?

On September 24, Randy, Jeffrey, and I headed to Dr. Cade's office for the initial TES session. The 'juice' was turned up significantly before Jeffrey responded to the electrical current with slight twitching in his legs. However, once he did respond (even if minimally), we managed to sing our way through the twenty-minute session quite effortlessly, thanks to the endless animals and contraptions Old MacDonald had acquired on his farm. That promising mission accomplished without interference from disaster, we headed home.

As soon as we pulled into the driveway, we spied a family of five deer by one of the big maple trees in the back—parents, two pre-teenish ones, and a baby one with spots.

After oohing at them for a few seconds, Randy looked down at Jeffrey and commented, "He's gurgly." I couldn't respond to that statement, as Jeffrey had been gurgly on a fairly regular basis for some time. I didn't need reminders. That evening I almost snapped when Randy, stuck with fixing dinner as usual, handed me a pan and told me it needed to be washed so he could use it, and I realized that my fuse was shorter than I thought—a whole lot shorter. Maybe there was no fuse at all any more. No matter that Randy had played dad and mom and breadwinner and maid and cook and chauffeur and errand boy for months and was also struggling to maintain composure and routine in a situation that was anything but normal.

After sloshing some soapy water around in the pan and placing Jeffrey in the stroller to continue the perpetual watch for distress, I went for a walk up and down our country road. Matthew, obviously concerned that I would head straight for the nearby river, asked if he could join me—for the walk, not the river. By the time we finished our therapy walk, Matthew and I had had the opportunity to talk about life in an adult world that seemed to make no sense at times, and I was feeling more human. More refreshed.

Hopefully, refreshed enough for whatever hit next.

Forty

September 26 began early in extraordinarily unfortunate form. After what seemed like only moments of precious sleep, I raised my head off the pillow and instantly experienced a searing muscle pull in my neck and shoulder. The pain was agonizing, but the tears were more from absolute frustration and disbelief that I had something else to contend with... as if I were looking for anything more.

Jeffrey had an appointment for his second round of TES, which I didn't want him to miss, so Randy drew taxi duties. Because of his ability to assume this and so many duties popping up, the purpose of the involuntary removal from his coaching job was beginning to soak in. Being his own boss afforded both Randy and me the luxury of flexibility and enabled him to participate fully in this assignment, despite sacrificing virtually all financial security. As Jeffrey matters had taken precedence over money matters, however, financial insecurity was irrelevant at the moment.

The second TES session for Jeffrey didn't proceed as easily as the first session. Our little guinea pig whimpered the entire time, despite my steady efforts to distract his attention by singing... which, granted, could have easily contributed to his discomfort. Dr. Cade expressed pleasant surprise that Jeffrey seemed to be responding noticeably so soon, but it was obvious he wasn't comfortable even with the same setting as before.

I hated that Jeffrey had to endure anything unpleasant, but I kept telling myself that maybe the TES could stimulate even a few muscles and grind the insidious muscle atrophy to a stall, if not a complete halt. As long as there was a remote chance that

TES might prove successful in holding this relentless disease at bay a little longer, we would just have to be in temporary discomfort together.

After a very long twenty-minute session, Jeffrey conked out in Randy's arms while I became the recipient of a major chiropractic adjustment, to me as luxurious as I envisioned a day at the spa. It was a welcomed opportunity to be out of mommy/nurse commission even briefly, as the stress and worry and emotional strain on my brain was a constant in life now.

And the day was young.

Forty-one

Upon leaving the doctor's office, we stopped by Wal-Mart for diapers. Jeffrey was still rendered temporarily unconscious from his latest round of TES, so I hurried inside while Randy drove around the parking lot to keep the air conditioner running in the sweltering summer heat. The errand was speedy because Jeffrey would surely wake up before too long, starving.

We pulled into our driveway at 1:25pm, several hours after Jeffrey, still sleeping, had last nursed. The PT (physical therapist) scheduled to fit him for an appropriate carseat pulled into the driveway right behind us, and I hopped out of the car to wave her on towards the front door. Within seconds, I turned back to unbuckle Jeffrey's seat, expecting him to be waking up and hungry.

He was waking up, all right, and turning blue. I snatched him up, rushed inside, and suctioned him without wasting a second, praying madly that it was not The Moment.

Jeffrey pinked up quickly and seemed quite unshaken. I was trembling and on the verge of losing the lunch I hadn't yet had, but I managed to hold on long enough to greet Susan, an unknown nurse from Home Health who appeared at the front door only minutes later. Meanwhile, the PT assessed that the carseat wouldn't work, so she hastily abandoned the scene of madness, leaving Susan alone in the nut ward with the head nut named Yours Truly.

I assumed Susan was the new nurse familiar with pediatrics that our regular home health nurse, Tonya, had mentioned, but Susan said she used to work for hospice. Oh. I then surmised that her hospice experience was the reason she was sent, but she said Tonya had a cold and didn't want to expose Jeffrey to the germs.

Within minutes, I learned that Susan's husband was the man I had heard about in Ashe County with SMA III. Susan was most compassionate, and I realized I was secretly relieved to have contact with a nurse familiar with hospice and, as a bonus, SMA, especially after the afternoon's potential crisis. I felt confident we would be doing a regular business with hospice soon. Very soon.

That night, Randy took Matthew to a high school football game, a weekly excursion Matthew gleefully anticipated every hour once the previous week's game ended. I was glad there was something fun in the routine to occupy their time, while I kept my eyes on Jeffrey and the clock the entire evening.

Jeffrey's breathing was heavier than usual that evening, and I tried to rationalize for my own benefit that it stemmed from exhaustion with the day, not with life itself. I found myself writing notes for Katie, my worthy assistant, in the event that notifying 9-1-1 became a necessity, and we practiced her end of the potential conversation. She was pleased as always to be of service in the name of Jeffrey, but I knew she was hoping to continue watching television as her personal escape from our real world.

The butterflies in my stomach and heart began performing acrobatics of unparalleled athleticism. I vowed to attune myself even more to any changes in Jeffrey that might signal the beginning of his transition to friendlier territory. And I prayed that I would not only recognize any changes but, more importantly, be able to accept them. It was another heavy-duty prayer request marathon.

There would be plenty more.

Forty-two

During the night, negligible as usual in the sleep department, Jeffrey began whimpering. I picked him up from his usual spot on the bed between Randy and me and, thinking he might be hungry, tried to nurse him. That wasn't what he wanted and he refused the offer; however, he seemed sufficiently comforted simply being held, so that's what I did. I observed instantly that his heavy breathing from earlier had returned, but it then began alternating with light breathing. Very light. And then the breaths simply ceased for an alarming, indeterminable amount of time before resuming. Back and forth and round and round, from heavy breaths to light ones to none at all.

Just when I convinced myself that this new occurrence was a(nother) truly significant challenge to my emotional stamina, Jeffrey opened his eyes as wide as possible and stared at me briefly before his eyes rolled back and stopped in a half-closed position. And he slept.

I didn't. My imagination zoomed further into overdrive, and I knew our journey must be coming to a close.

But wait—I wasn't ready! Not that a parent could ever be adequately prepared to say good-by to his child permanently, but this was just too soon. There were so many things left to do… like figuring out how we would muster the emotional fortitude to let Jeffrey go.

After an hour of watching his unsettling pattern of breathing but reasonably assured that he was again sleeping peacefully, I carefully placed him back on his pillow between Randy and me, staring at him as if willing him not to go. And praying that God would see things my way… just a little while longer.

At least until Dorothy returned from Oz with a big basket of Courage.

Forty-three

I eventually drifted off to sleep from sheer exhaustion. Early in the morning, Jeffrey was awake, smiling, and hungry! The power of prayer was once again confirmed, and I felt confident I could tackle the crammed menu of tasks for the day.

Jeffrey was happy and comfortable only in my lap, so we spent the day in our ragged-but-comfy overstuffed Jeffrey chair. While I didn't accomplish a thing in the physical sense, I was able to evaluate our situation and ponder that maybe it was time to abandon the chaos of the medical regimen, the results of which were completely unknown at best. I had prayed often that God would provide us with the wisdom to make tough decisions, presuming foolishly that there would be easy ones. I felt time had come for me to be a mama, although it would be impossible to sever my nurse ties completely, and for Jeffrey to be a baby rather than a guinea pig. Despite my gut feeling, I wavered momentarily over the notion to abort his treatment, hoping and praying my instinct was headed in the right direction.

I shared my thoughts with Randy; he also seemed resigned to the fact that the end of our assignment was approaching and that we might as well enjoy what we could. *Enjoy.* I couldn't imagine using that word again.

That night, Katie cried with a sore throat, Matthew needed his inhaler, and my head pounded. Without a word, Randy left the house to hike up the little mountain, no doubt scoping out the road diligently being carved out to transport Jeffrey some day to his resting spot on top. I figured he was also stocking up on some spiritual vibes in the process and hoped he would bring some back for me.

I looked on the previous night's events as a rehearsal, as Duffy's death had been, for the main event. As the old adage goes, practice makes perfect. Except that with no script in our hands, we wouldn't know if we were in rehearsal or the real performance until the curtain closed a final time.

I wasn't sure how many more rehearsals it would take for us to get it right, or how many more we could endure.

And that included Jeffrey.

Forty-four

September 28 was, like so many other days in our Jeffrey journey, eventful. I had to suction Jeffrey not only before breakfast, but during his tub time, too, as he threatened to turn blue. The tears flowed for us all; even without sharing words, we seemed to believe collectively that our time with Jeffrey was drawing to a close.

As soon as Randy left to pick Katie up from a birthday party, Jeffrey's breathing became erratic again, the periods of shallow breathing alternating with none at all. My attention shifted from Jeffrey to the clock and back. I prayed that his breathing would again become as steady and reliable as the clock's ticking and hoped that the clock wasn't in danger of stopping. In his usual fashion, Jeffrey not only held on until Randy and Katie returned, he began smiling and babbling, louder than ever! I wondered what he was trying to tell us.

Randy made a rather secretive phone call to someone he later reluctantly identified, upon my questioning, as Gary of Badger Funeral Home. It never ceased to amaze me how capably and *willingly* Randy managed phone conversations. To have been able to share the diagnosis and death sentence with family members before we could absorb it ourselves, and now to discuss arrangements that concerned placing our baby's body in a casket? That was way out of my league.

Gary explained to Randy that since the death of a baby was so traumatic, their Cherub Service took care of the financial aspects of the arrangements when it concerned an infant. While I hadn't given any thought to the financial aspects of funeral planning (primarily because giving thought to a funeral itself was miserable), I was relieved not to have to add it to the list. Earth angels continued scrambling on our behalf.

Mom and Dad came over later with a carseat, but I didn't think it would work. I also didn't think it mattered, anyway, as I couldn't fathom taking Jeffrey anywhere again. Doctors were now out, and he was becoming increasingly dependent on my lap and in the Jeffrey chair, in particular, for comfort and safety and preparation for his own assignment. The final one.

Jeffrey had nursed only on his right side for a few days, resulting in a bit of lopsidedness on my part, though it hardly hampered my lumpy physique. I was grateful he found comfort in some position. When I tried to shift him around to offer him a change of scenery, he let me know without hesitation that he had already seen enough.

He knew what he wanted. And how to get it.

A weird sense of acceptance crept into my psyche, stemming from the increased conviction that Jeffrey knew exactly what was happening. So when Matthew brought up some valid questions, from "What if something happens and we're at school?" to "What (equipment) will we get rid of first?," I responded in a calm, rational, upbeat, and confident manner.

I'd collect the Oscar on my way to the rubber room.

Forty-five

Katie coughed all night, so I didn't even attempt to wake her for school the following morning. Matthew called Papa to come get him for school so I could stay with Jeffrey and Katie, but the volcano in his stomach convinced him that going to school probably wasn't a wise move after all. As our neighbor carpooler was also sick, I figured the school folks would assume something had happened.

Something did happen.

Jeffrey awoke and cooed, "Uh-oh!" While he was probably forewarning us of the day's events, I looked on it as another miracle, another boost to our emotional systems, ammo for what lay ahead.

Matthew and Katie were in a full-fledged discussion mode, so I decided to read aloud from the Bible about Job, assuring them and reminding myself that substantial obstacles in life have fallen obtrusively into the paths of other good folks since ancient times. After a few minutes and a few Job disasters later, Matthew commented, "That sounds like us."

Poor Job. Poor us.

Later in the day, tears fell at everything I observed—the clouds floating across the sky, the neighbor cows' antics (like standing and chewing), Nellie's sleeping, Randy, Matthew, Katie, Jeffrey. I realized I had no clue as to the day or date, as they had been running into each other too long. The concept of time was a blur. Life in general was a blur.

Our predicament was not.

Forty-six

Jeffrey had an exceptionally easy time on September 30, and yet I bawled almost all day long. I had no idea why, either, unless the stress toxins were out of control. Maybe it was relief that he was doing so well.

Or it could easily have been the emotional exhaustion of continuously preparing for one end of the spectrum of his existence and then being yanked to the opposite end and back again... the yo-yo effect. It didn't seem to matter whether we were preparing 'for better' or 'for worse'—the certainty of what was coming combined with the uncertainty of knowing when or how was driving us all to the wacky ward. I would be the first one to the door... and probably pushed in. I really needed to pack.

Knowing I would have to face it some time, I attempted feebly to organize the obituary information, but it was simply unbearable. The tears were relentless, and I wondered—as I had numerous times before—why *we* were the ones having to make out a death notice for our baby, why *we* were the ones going through such hell, why *we* were losing our baby... especially when we still hadn't quite figured out how he came to be.

Surprisingly, I'd never considered myself angry at God, but my confusion at this devastating assignment defied comprehension. I felt certain that some day we'd know the answers, but that it might not be during our earth time. I hoped I had the patience—and sanity—to wait.

Giving up on the obituary, I moved on to my next dreaded task, that of choosing a going-away outfit. Another migraine moment. Jeffrey seemed amused by his solo fashion show, smiling and babbling especially animatedly when I finally selected an outfit with *Baby pandas like to play* on the front. His panda-loving cousin, Bethany, had brought it to him. It was a special outfit because of that, and I knew he'd be doing a lot of playing soon.

Mission accomplished, Jeffrey then moved his arm at the shoulder, something he had never done. Was I imagining it? Was he waving good-bye, or was I witnessing another tiny miracle of improvement? I knew that if I wasn't committed soon, that in itself would be a miracle. A big one.

With Jeffrey feeling so good, I once again considered taking him to Asheville for consultation with a pulmonologist currently treating another child with SMA, also from Cary, North Carolina (home of my closest online angel and president of the proposed NC Chapter of FSMA, Cindy). The evaluation would determine whether or not Jeffrey could benefit not only from BiPAP—simply, a type of assisted-breathing machine—but also from Gabapentin, a drug typically used for patients with ALS.

The notion of taking Jeffrey three hours from home on what I already considered borrowed time and a last-ditch effort was frightening, and yet so was the thought of not trying it if it could be done without distressing him. I craved reassurance that we were employing absolutely any and every possible tactic that might thwart the degeneration, and we would never know if we didn't ask.

An entire day of contemplation provided no answers. Jeffrey put his paci in his mouth with his left hand, which was a first, but he also had increased difficulty nursing, latching on and sucking. I rationalized that the late hour might have something to do with it, but I didn't know. Meanwhile, Matthew and Katie began beefing up the questions and expressing their fear that something would happen to Jeffrey while they were at school. My answer to them was simple and familiar: "Let's pray."

I was beginning to feel qualified to take over the pulpit... as Preacher Looney Toon.

Forty-seven

By October, I made sure Matthew and Katie said good-bye to Jeffrey and hugged him each morning before they left for the safety and sanity of school. Katie's class had a field trip to Winston-Salem on the first day of the month. I was happy she would have a distraction of enjoyment, but it took a concerted effort to contain myself from worrying that something might happen while she was gone. What would we do if it did? If 'something' happened, we couldn't keep Jeffrey at home until Katie returned, and yet I couldn't imagine having to take her to the funeral home to see his body. The prayers intensified that we would be at home, together, when the end came.

Jeffrey's irregular breathing, from fast to shallow to nothing for what seemed like hours, kept me spellbound. He had a few fussy episodes, but he also smiled and jabbered in a rather distractive manner, as if talking to the angels. Making plans.

By noon, I realized just how dependent I had become on clocks, observing how many hours, minutes, and seconds were left before each family member returned home. While I'd always depended on clocks, I now felt like an addict of sorts. Or a hostage.

During the afternoon, Jeffrey mostly slept in my lap but cried out on occasion. Was he uncomfortable? Was he ready to go? Did he want to stay? Was he hearing instructions from Above that were upsetting (perhaps that he couldn't leave just yet?)? Bad dream? I also noticed his nostrils flaring—that was something new, and I was quite sure not good, as I'd read it meant a struggle for oxygen.

His breathing continued erratically, his eyes seemingly malfunctioned at half-mast. I found myself mumbling permission for him to go on, to accompany the angels who seemed to be drawing him closer. To say that was excruciating is a gross understatement, but desperate times called for desperate measures. I couldn't know that even more desperate times were in the works.

At that precise moment, Jeffrey woke up, smiled like crazy, and began babbling at breakneck speed. Did offering permission ease the load for him in some way? What did he know, and what was he trying to tell me?

I wondered if maybe the undeniably pure joy illuminating from babies and children affected by SMA stemmed from their knowledge of what lay ahead in God's plans. Maybe the apparent frustration for them on occasion was the inability to convey the 'angel' understanding, their very essence, to those of us still grounded firmly in the earthling phase. Who knew? Who was even privy to know?

Obviously, not I.

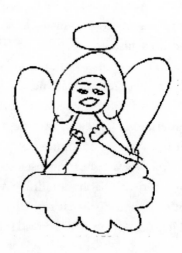

Forty-eight

On October 2, Jeffrey enjoyed a good morning and a great afternoon. About the time I began reflecting (cautiously) on just how well the day had gone so far, the mail arrived with the requested packet of information concerning the pulmonologist in Asheville, Dr. Brown*. I read the report of the trials with Gabapentin and the use of BiPAP, witnessed the exuberance of Jeffrey's bright eyes and radiant smile (*Go for it, Mama!*), and decided that that was the sign I'd been waiting for. I called the doctor's office immediately and was told to bring Jeffrey in on Monday, October 6.

With the decision to investigate BiPAP and Gabapentin made and appointment scheduled, I relaxed more the rest of the day than I had since the time prior to the diagnosis nearly three months before. The optimism must have been contagious, as even our stoic Matthew began cracking jokes. What a grand feeling it was to be laughing and feeling hopeful again!

To add to the upbeat atmosphere, a mom called from Lenoir after reading my letter about Jeffrey in the paper. She had a 16-year old daughter with Type 1, an honor student, content with her life. More sparks of hope and confidence that this was a purposeful mission.

Tonya, our home health nurse, came on October 3, another good day for our little guy. She didn't bring scales on that visit, but it didn't matter. We were going to Asheville in three days, and I knew Jeffrey would be weighed and measured then. Besides, I didn't want to know if there had been additional weight loss as a result of diminishing muscle mass. Our formerly chubby dumpling was beginning to look long and lean, a body type utterly foreign to both sides of our family.

Randy and Matthew prepared for their high school football excursion that evening. As they were leaving, Katie hollered to Matthew, "You take the inhaler to the game, 'cause we can just call Rescue 9-1-1 from here."

I hoped that was not premonition on Katie's part and that we could squeak by without the services of the inhaler or 'Rescue 9-1-1' for just a little longer.

Forty-nine

It took until the fifth day of the month for it to register that it had become October. My concept of time had been completely warped, if present at all, for months. Time, like sleep and sanity and everything else, had acquired new interpretation long ago.

Jeffrey stayed awake and alert for almost five hours, so I grabbed the opportunity and bathed him in the big tub. He loved water and the ability it gave him to move freely, and this time was no exception. He cooed, waving his forearms and sliding his legs back and forth gleefully and effortlessly, further proof to me that our upcoming trip was the right move in this assignment chock full of critical decisions.

Paul and Jaymie came to visit, no doubt thinking, after recent events, that it might be their last opportunity to see Jeffrey. Randy went up the mountain to check the progress of our new Jeffrey road, then he went up later with Matthew. Trooper that she was, Nellie trotted beside Randy both times, providing vital companionship for him in my absence.

I was curious to see what had been done with the road that would some day guide us to Jeffrey's resting spot on the top of the mountain, but I could wait for the reason it was being done. The day was gorgeous, and I felt almost confident that it would be an uneventful one. When I calculated only 24 hours and 45 minutes left before our appointment in Asheville, I felt another surge of hope that our luck and our lives had shifted for the better. It was a joyous feeling!

And it wouldn't last.

Fifty

On the morning of October 6, a day I hadn't been so sure we'd share with Jeffrey, we gathered up the necessities for our trip to Asheville and the pulmonologist: suction machine, suction bulb, diapers, water, bottle warmer, empty bottle for pumping, pillow, map, notes, directions, Jeffrey, and whatever remnants of lucidity, sanity, and hope we could scrounge up. We were eager to leave, anxious about the trip, and optimistic about what we'd learn from Dr. Brown.

After getting Matthew and Katie squared away with Nana and Papa for the day, we headed out for our three-hour drive, Jeffrey in his carseat and me beside him in the back seat. We hadn't gone two miles from home before he needed to be suctioned. That was not a good sign, but I was ready and cranked the suction machine into action.

There was too little *oomph* on the battery pack to be useful, though, so we hastily made the decision to return home, where I could suction Jeffrey with the benefit of an electrical outlet. Meanwhile, Randy would try to track down an adapter for the car that would enable us to reach Asheville, where we'd be in competent hands for whatever crisis materialized (if we'd only known…).

While I suctioned Jeffrey, Randy did locate an adapter at Radio Shack in Boone, about thirty miles from us and right on the way to Asheville. That was a welcomed break, so things were back to looking up! We would just swing by the store at the mall, pick up the adapter, and head on to Asheville. We weren't running late—yet—but we no longer had any time to spare.

When the suctioning was completed, we were off to Boone.

This time, the pillow was in my lap, and Jeffrey was lying down on it, facing me. I prayed we'd reach Asheville without additional glitches, rationalizing that he was surely better off in my lap without a seat belt than upright and buckled in his carseat, struggling to swallow with progressively inadequate swallowing muscles. Still, I hoped we wouldn't draw attention to ourselves in view of anyone in a uniform and a foul mood.

When we reached the mall, I removed the cannula (tubing) so Randy could carry the machine inside to verify the adapter's compatibility without having to worry about the cannula's unraveling all over the floor. He rushed inside and back out with the proper adapter, and we were once again on the road to Asheville.

Foresight would have headed us back home.

Fifty-one

The remainder of the ride to Asheville, with Jeffrey cozy on his pillow, was uneventful, except for the vibrant colors along the way. The trees, in their autumn finery, were simply breathtaking, reminding me why I had always considered fall my favorite season, at least until spring arrived. This year, I had missed out on the splendor even in our own backyard.

We arrived at Dr. Brown's office and completed the requisite forms. It wasn't long before we were ushered back to the room by a nice nurse for the ritual of undressing Jeffrey, then measuring (off the chart, as usual, at 28 inches) and weighing him. We were pleased to see he'd gained a quarter ounce to almost fifteen pounds! His weight was significantly below normal compared to his length because of the lack of muscle mass, so even a hint of weight gain, or no weight loss, was celebrated.

Afterwards, the nurse carefully placed Jeffrey on the exam table, where he could coo and admire the cute baby in the wall mirror. And he did! Despite his likely premature death sentence from SMA, he possessed an extraordinarily cheery disposition.

Dr. Brown came into the room after just a few minutes' wait on our part. Patiently and with what appeared to be genuine interest and concern, he asked what we were hoping to achieve (*other than saving our baby's life, you mean?*). I explained that we'd heard he was using Gabapentin on another SMA baby with seemingly good results, and we wanted to see if Jeffrey might be a good candidate for the drug. We also desired to learn if the use of BiPAP would provide sufficient rest for him at nighttime in the rigorous process to which most of us pay no attention... breathing.

He nodded understandingly and then brought up, out of

left field, his desire to first try the mechanical In-Exsufflator on Jeffrey. This was a machine designed to provide coughing assistance for those whose muscles are too weak to produce an independent, spontaneous cough. I'd read about the machine and its benefits in clearing the lungs of harbored gunk, but I mentioned to Dr. Brown that I'd understood it was for those old enough to follow directions and cough on command. His response was, "It helps, but it's not necessary."

Famous last words.

He was thoughtful enough to explain that the process would freak Jeffrey out, as the machine's purpose was to externally simulate a cough in its quest to clear out excessive mucous. The machine would blow air into Jeffrey's lungs, then quickly suck it out. I tried to block out the vision of the anticipated effect, figuring that he with the official medical degree knew what he was doing. Hoping so, anyway, as our original intentions for being there had apparently been temporarily shelved while we played his game.

Dr. Brown left the room and returned in a few minutes, lugging with him the ominous-looking machine. He plugged it in, placed the mask on Jeffrey's face, and turned it on, creating a deadly noise as he began the procedure. Jeffrey's eyes expressed the absolute terror he must have felt when the first 'cough' occurred. It was an expression immediately mirrored in Randy's face and in mine. It was excruciating to watch, and I felt I had betrayed Jeffrey completely.

When I thought that was it—for the treatment, for Jeffrey's trust in us, for what was left of my waning mental and emotional state—Dr. Brown instructed me to do it so I'd know how.

Hesitating, while telling myself repeatedly that it was for Jeffrey's benefit, I turned the machine on and immediately felt as if I were in command of the electric chair, knowingly frying an innocent person. Even more horrifying... the innocent person was my own child. Jeffrey's eyes looked as if they would burst out of their sockets with fright and disbelief, and ours were no better. Maybe worse, as we were the parents, the ones assigned the responsibility of keeping our children safe from harm.

Thankfully, the experiment ended quickly, and Dr. Brown turned the monster box off. I had already decided I wasn't about to haul that bright idea home and was eager to get to the real reason for our being there, thankful we had survived the nightmare of the past few minutes.

It wasn't over, though. It was just beginning.

Another beginning of the end.

Fifty-two

When Dr. Brown checked Jeffrey's lungs upon conclusion of the agonizing demonstration, he commented, "He sounds a little gurgly. Let's try it again to try to get that out." On went the machine, and another torturous treatment began. This time, though, Jeffrey immediately became limp and began turning blue. He was in respiratory arrest! We were zapped smack dab into the middle of a horrific nightmare within a horrific nightmare, and it only intensified when Randy and I realized there was no suction machine in the office, of a pulmonologist, in whose care we had placed our baby! There was no oxygen in sight, either, which made the entire ordeal even more unbelievable.

Randy was instantly jolted into a functioning capacity and rushed to the car to get our suction machine. Before he had time to return, I realized with a sickening horror that I hadn't replaced the cannula I'd removed at the mall. In the meantime, Dr. Brown began mouth-to-mouth resuscitation in his quest to revive our baby, who had been in his care all of ten minutes. I agonized over leaving Jeffrey for even a moment, but the suction machine was critical; I had to believe I would return in time. As Randy raced back into the room with the machine, I then sprinted urgently amid the now-curious and increasingly wary patients in the waiting room to retrieve the cannula from the car.

I flew back with the cannula to find the nurse rolling out their cannula supply pack and gawked in disturbing disbelief at what looked like a thousand choices. I feared she would never find the right size, which Dr. Brown felt should be smaller than the one we used at home and held, terrified, in our hands.

In unbelievably surreal slow motion, the EMTs reported for disaster duty as Jeffrey began pinking back up. They seemed to be in no recognizable state of emergency whatsoever, which did nothing to assuage my personal state of panic. Wisely, though, they put me on the stretcher first before placing Jeffrey in my lap, with my hand holding the oxygen mask over his nose and both of us in pure shock. Poor Randy was left on his own to follow the ambulance in our car. I hoped and prayed he would be able to keep up with what was sure to be a speedy trip to the emergency room, as I didn't see how he could possibly still be in possession of enough sense to find the way himself.

The only bit of good fortune in the cruel turn of events was that the hospital was located just across the parking lot from the office, so I imagine the ride was brief. It didn't feel brief, however, as the speed of the rescue vehicle seemed to max out at a whopping two miles per hour.

Once we reached the emergency room and Jeffrey was placed carefully on the exam table, he promptly went into respiratory arrest for the second time. Endless ER scenes from television popped into my consciousness. This time, however, the doctors, nurses, and crisis were real, and the patient was our precious baby. There was also no guarantee that the crisis would be resolved soon or that the ending would be happy.

Watching various staff members trying to revive Jeffrey by jamming tubes down his throat and knowing that he must be yearning to make his permanent escape was more than I could stand, and I had a terrifyingly realistic, split-second, spontaneous image of my rescuing him... by suffocating him with a pillow.

Anything to free him from this nightmare.

With that unfathomable thought, I knew I was beyond ready for my own cubby in the looney bin, packed or not. And throw away the key. Please.

At the peak of my fast-approaching lunacy in its most complete form, I was called out of the ER to handle paperwork. I figured the hospital personnel were mainly afraid Jeffrey was going to die in the ER, and they didn't want a maternal maniac in there. I wasn't sure any of the information I offered was correct, but that was hardly a priority at the moment. When the hospital folks were satisfied I had provided at least the bulk of the necessary information, Randy returned from the ER with a report that Jeffrey was okay, relatively speaking, and he and I were then whisked away to talk to the chaplain and expose our inner souls.

There wasn't much exposing on our end, as I was sobbing, and Randy teetered on the brink. I had thought in the very beginning of our Jeffrey journey that the donation of Jeffrey's organs would be a generous, uplifting idea; however, upon hearing that the patient had to be kept dependent on machines until the organs were removed, I decided, admittedly selfishly, that I'd rather have him at home when the end came.

Now I wondered what God's plans were. I certainly wasn't able to follow His train of thought. Was this agonizing subplot an opportunity to share Jeffrey in another way? To keep at least part of him here in the earthly sense?

I didn't want to make any decisions; I just wanted to go home—with Jeffrey—where we all belonged.

DEAR GOD, I KNOW YOU'RE THERE. I KNOW YOU'RE *HERE*. HELP US.

PLEASE...

Fifty-three

Countless blurred minutes with the chaplain lapsed before Randy and I were finally allowed to return to Jeffrey in the emergency room, where I was asked to hold him almost as soon as we walked into his area. I prayed the request wasn't nearly as ominous as it sounded and was overwhelmed with relief to see that our little guy looked quite calm... and was still breathing. The ER staff and Dr. Brown, who had legitimately earned his pallor, proceeded to explain the options to us (in essence, BiPAP or nothing) and asked what we wanted to do.

We decided to proceed with overnight BiPAP for the sole purpose of stabilizing Jeffrey enough to go home the next day. At the rate we were going, I was convinced we had been hurled against our will into a game of Russian roulette, and the click of the trigger determined whether the medical profession would help us get Jeffrey home... or kill him in the process.

With the decision made, the next move was to transfer Jeffrey to PICU (Pediatric ICU), so off we went. Following a nurse leading the way, I held Jeffrey and *walked*, while someone in a white coat followed behind me, pulling the oxygen tank... possibly for me. I thought that was mighty considerate of him but wondered just how competent those folks could be if they were letting me (or making me) walk to the elevator and up to PICU on spaghetti legs—carrying precious cargo in my arms—after all we'd just been through. Were they crazy (Door #1) or just incompetent (Door #2)? Swell choices.

Sorry, time's up. You lose.

Numbness and shock, both effective anesthetics, and a determination to take Jeffrey home the following day propelled me all the way to his room. Fortunately, there was no conversation from anyone to disturb my focus. Not that it could have been disturbed.

When we reached our new room, a kind nurse took Jeffrey from me and gently placed him on the giant bed. As our tiny warrior was surrounded by nurses who seemed both caring and competent, Randy left for a few minutes, probably to fortify himself somehow for whatever was coming next.

What came next, while he was still out of the room, was another episode of respiratory arrest, and the tears gushed... again. For the first time, I was angry at God and screamed silently—*WHAT ARE YOU DOING HERE?* **ARE** *YOU HERE? WHY ARE YOU PUTTING JEFFREY THROUGH THIS? WHAT HAVE WE DONE TO DESERVE THIS? WHAT HAS* **HE** *DONE TO DESERVE THIS?*

A wonderful big black nurse named Mary must have been assigned as our angel-on-call at that moment, proving once again that God hadn't abandoned us, although it may have seemed that way at times. Her presence was instantly of great comfort, despite the fact that she didn't provide any words of wisdom or answers to my pleas to God.

I decided it must be a miserable job to have nothing to offer but a hug when the end of life for a loved one, particularly a child, seemed inevitable; however, no gauge can measure the worth of a hug. I gratefully absorbed the warmth, comfort, and security of Mary's understanding arms and, rejuvenated to some extent by her graciously loving spirit, shared another hug with Randy when he returned to the room for whatever came next.

For better, for worse...

Fifty-four

With the help of the nurse angels, Jeffrey once again pinked up and was hooked up to the BiPAP. Somehow he had enough spunk left to protest the placement of another mask on his face and the efforts of the machine itself to conserve energy he expended just to breathe. After twenty minutes of balking, however, he conked out for several hours, allowing the machine to regulate his breathing and provide him with a long-overdue break from the trauma of life.

I kept my eyes glued to him, disturbed somewhat about his dry lips and bubbly mouth but confident I could manage vaseline and a kleenex. I just wanted his condition to improve enough for the trip back home.

As with the diagnosis hospital stay, there were wires to monitor oxygen saturation levels, heart rate, and respiratory rate. An IV was placed in his left knee for potential emergencies, nurses constantly checked or requested something (blood pressure, IV, monitors, diapers, blood), and there was a steady stream of chest PT (pounding), suctioning, and consultations.

By then, my brain fuzz was totally and possibly irreversibly disheveled, but I was alert and focused enough to continue the vigil. At least this room had a relatively comfortable rocker, and we were right across the hall from the nurses' station. I considered the proximity a reward for surviving the consultation-that-wasn't rather than dwelling on the likelihood that we would need attention in a moment's notice.

I learned from two nurses on separate occasions that the In-Ex-sufflator had a nickname around the halls... The Suffocator. I had read about too many positive attributes of the machine for older children and adults to dismiss its usefulness in the world of SMA, but my stomach lurched at its role in our current dilemma.

Paul called the hospital that evening and told Randy he was coming to Asheville to follow us home the next day, whether I wanted him to or not. I was batty but not stupid; his presence as a competent member of the medical profession and as a brother were welcomed more than he knew. By that time, I gladly took what I could get, and I knew Randy was equally grateful for additional relief and support. Paul's presence would also enable at least one of us to grab a few moments of the sleep we desperately needed.

Jeffrey awoke several hours later in a state of confusion, but he nursed readily and snuggled up in safety from the evil-doers and all that they would do if he weren't glued to his mama. I wished I could keep him from all of them and just go home.

The nurse on duty, also named Helen, was wonderful, and when she saw how cozy her little patient was in my lap, she didn't insist on whisking him back to BiPAP prison. He lingered contentedly in my lap several more hours until the respiratory therapist (RT) came in, miffed because Jeffrey was still not hooked up to the machine. I reluctantly placed him in the bed for incarceration, where his balking in Round Two lasted only about five minutes before he fell fast asleep. At some point Paul arrived, and I knew then that we'd make it home, anyway. What happened once we arrived would be another chapter, one I'd tackle when we came to it.

Jeffrey slept well, but he was more than ready to be released from his BiPAP confinement when his nap ended. The RT thought he needed to stay on a little while longer, though, and for the first time since the diagnosis testing ordeal, I saw tears trickling from both of his eyes. That meant enough in my opinion, which I shared distinctly with the RT, and she reluctantly agreed to take him off.

131

Once again, he relaxed in my arms, nursing easily despite the wires monitoring his every move, and the tubing for the blow-by oxygen for comfort that I controlled to avoid a nasal tube placement. My heartfelt prayers for a safe return home continued, and I graciously accepted the minutes that passed without incidence as the answer that we would, indeed, make it home with Jeffrey.

Much too soon, the RT returned to hook Jeffrey up to the BiPAP machine for the third time. His eyes were wide with apprehension as she loomed over the bed, and the tears started again. An absolutely eternal fifteen minutes passed after she hooked him up before I said firmly, "He doesn't like it. Take it off." She sighed, probably mumbling under her breath about the ignorance of some parents, but she removed it, anyway.

She was no dummy. I doubt I would have pushed the matter had I thought we had a long trial period to work with, but I felt sure we didn't. Away from the BiPAP, Jeffrey was safe with Randy, Paul, and me and would stay that way until we left the hospital insanity. For safety. For Matthew and Katie.

For home.

For whatever.

Fifty-five

The BiPAP experiment was deemed enough of a success the next morning for Jeffrey to go home (thank You, dear Father). The morning was spent in discussion of the problem that had rendered us overnighters—possibly a collapsed lung or too much gunk in the lung—and the consideration of a bronchoscopy, a technique using a lighted instrument to view the airways, to see for sure. Dr. Brown, who initiated the matter of the invasive procedure, favored it with enthusiasm, but the intensivist, whatever that was, thought the procedure might be too much for Jeffrey. End of discussion. I appreciated the intensivist's honesty and didn't know if I could trust Dr. Brown's judgment for anything at that point.

Dr. Brown continued his earlier discussion of placement of an NJ feeding tube (from the nose to the small intestine) in Jeffrey. After he completed the description of the procedure, which even he admitted was uncomfortable, he might as well have been talking to the bed rail. I was through listening. It sounded like more agony for Jeffrey, and since he seemed to be nursing just fine and had had more than his share of misery already, thanks to a handful of medical geniuses, I knew we wouldn't go through with it. It seemed quite obvious to me that Jeffrey would be a high-risk candidate for any sort of surgical procedure at that point.

In addition, Dr. Brown had the audacity to bring up a place for the In-Exsufflator in Jeffrey's treatment and that he'd like to see him in two weeks for serious discussion of that and placement of the NJ tube.

I had had enough rejuvenation of a few senses to recognize a joker/lunatic/idiot when I saw one. And one was occupying the chair across from me. I nodded slightly, fearing we wouldn't be released if we didn't agree to meet his demands. He didn't have to know that the nod meant something else.

Like hell we'll be back.

Throughout the course of the morning, I asked the doctors and nurses if they thought Jeffrey could handle the upcoming ride home, and the answer was a resounding, "Oh, yes!" He would need ready access to oxygen and probably a good deal of suctioning on the way home... both manageable and anticipated.

The equipment deemed essential for the ride was gathered up for us: a BiPAP machine (though I felt sure we'd never use it), the portable oxygen canisters and tubing, the suctioning machine we'd brought from home, and a back-up suctioning machine from the hospital. All of these would remain at home upon our arrival, converting our mini house into a mini medical facility.

When I asked, wearily and warily, for the umpteenth time about the ride home and repeated the rather significant information that we lived three hours away, the staff replied in unison, "Oh."

That was not what I wanted to hear. They said then that the oxygen canister would not be enough for the ride, so how about a nasal cannula for Jeffrey? I replied that they needed to find something else, as nothing was going down his nose. They obediently obliged, bringing back a standard Dixie cup for the end of the tubing to distribute the oxygen on a blow-by basis. It would probably be assigned a ridiculous price on the bill I silently dared them to send, but I didn't care. Getting home was the focus of the moment.

While I suctioned Jeffrey one last time before our departure, two nurses worked to dislodge the IV installed in his knee. I glanced in their direction, horrified to see that it resembled an enormous, mutant steel nail, and for the first time, I was truly appreciative of the distraction my suctioning duties provided.

Poor baby. I had no idea how he would ever forgive us for this entire fiasco but knew it wouldn't happen again. No more guinea pig time for any of us. This time, enough was more than enough.

The medical supplies were loaded up, and I was handed a packet of papers which included instructions on how to dial 9-1-1 should Jeffrey stop breathing. I fought the urge to file them right then, deciding that I'd better wait until I got home and out of sight to ditch them appropriately. No way would I try to bring Jeffrey back to his private hell on earth whenever an opportunity to escape was provided by the One in charge.

And I felt confident that Opportunity would come knocking very soon.

Fifty-six

The interior of the car was morphed into a sort of hospital supply company on wheels, and Jeffrey and I squeezed into our tiny spot for the long ride. Our little center of attention was placed gently on his pillow in my lap and Paul prepared to follow behind in his own vehicle. The staff was no doubt relieved to see us headed on our way and, I felt sure, genuinely hoping for an uneventful trip. I asked for prayers from them for our journey home and prayed nonstop myself that we would make it all the way. Even if we just reached the driveway before the onset of another and possibly final catastrophe, at least we would all be together again.

The Dixie cup contraption was put to use almost as soon as the door was shut, allowing blow-by the oxygen to ease Jeffrey's breathing… hopefully for the duration of the ride home. It did.

Our trusty old house popped into view in early evening, and what a beautiful sight it was! My folks were already there with Matthew and Katie, along with the representative from a pediatric medical supply company. She had come to deliver an oxygenator and an additional portable oxygen canister.

The oxygenator removed the nitrogen from the surrounding (room) air, leaving mostly oxygen, and included a fifty-foot piece of tubing which extended sufficiently all over our compact house. The machine utilized the blow-by method of providing oxygen to Jeffrey as needed to keep him comfortable and would stay on until he didn't need it anymore. At that point, our assignment would most likely be over.

Randy called Dr. Brown to let him know we had reached friendly territory without crisis; he seemed glad to hear it, if a bit surprised. The hospital called later to inform us that neither Randy nor I had signed the discharge papers. Oops. I feared momentarily it was a sign that something else unpleasant lurked around the corner, but just as quickly deemed it a fitting end to the latest three-ring hoopla.

After making sure everyone was settled, Randy walked to the mountain top on the new Jeffrey road to check on its progress. The road was much more than a simple clearing of trees to accommodate transportation. Randy reminded me of the significant events on mountaintops reported in the Bible, with Jesus at the helm. It was fitting that we had our own little mountain, and one with a cemetery on top; another major event was about to occur, and both the mountaintop and Jesus would play prominent roles.

The road would provide us with a physical link from Jeffrey's spot in his earthly home to his upcoming resting spot, a site so close to heaven, we could reach for the very stars that would soon welcome him Home. Symbolically, the road would enable us to remain connected with our special little guy in a different way. I grabbed for straws of anything positive as an adhesive for my frayed emotional wiring. Super Glue and duct tape together would not begin to do the trick. Straws, maybe.

Randy came back down fairly quickly, reporting that Toby, another of our miracle workers, had been working diligently on the Jeffrey road and that it was almost finished.

Good thing.

Fifty-seven

Our first night back home was a good, blissfully uninterrupted one for Jeffrey, but he slept fitfully throughout the following day, appeased by nothing but my lap. I eagerly obliged and attempted to doze as he did. He was duly exhausted from the madness in Asheville; I wondered if he wasn't feeling good or if he was ready to leave this nuthouse altogether. I certainly couldn't blame him for seeking safer grounds, where those we envisioned in white were called angels.

Tonya, our nurse angel, made her regular home health visit and cried most of the time, as she had already heard about the ordeal. She said the nurse who had contacted her from the hospital told her I was not being realistic about the likely outcome of what we were dealing with. Tonya assured her that I was most realistic about what was coming. Jeepers, it had only been our target of focus and prayer for three months.

The hospital nurse's 'observation' was as absurd as what another nurse had charted immediately after the diagnosis: *Mother upset and crying.* I wasn't sure what reaction she had expected or regarded as normal or acceptable; I certainly couldn't imagine any other. Maybe she had simply stood too close to Dr. Doom.

After checking Jeffrey and observing his alarmingly lethargic condition, Tonya very gently suggested that maybe it was time for her to contact hospice. I agreed. Jeffrey had been zapped in a big way this time, and I wasn't sure he would be able to pull out of the current funk. I wondered if he wanted to pull out of it… or, even more alarmingly, if I wanted him to. Whereas he had flitted from mostly pure joy and contentment (or at least comfort) to only minimal discomfort before the eventful non-

138

consultation in Asheville, I didn't know if he could flit anymore. Maybe his earthly wings had been clipped, readying him for angel wings. Only God knew, and He didn't seem to be talking… to me, anyway.

A nurse from hospice called later in the day to tell me that several staff members would come out to the house the following day. A part of me felt relief, but a bigger part of me was overcome with sickening anticipation at the reason for the impending visit.

Increasingly, I felt as if my own earthly wings were disintegrating.

Only there were no angel wings waiting for me.

Fifty-eight

Octber 9... Hospice Day. Two nurses and a social worker from hospice came and stayed three hours. Mary, a nurse, began by saying—carefully and quietly—that they were all moms, that Jeffrey was their youngest client ever, and that they would be learning from me. In the throes of full-fledged exhaustion, I wasn't overly comforted to hear that I would be leading another pack, but I understood it and appreciated their apparent willingness to listen to me. I hoped they would have more to hear than the shattering of my heart.

Mary gently examined Jeffrey, checking vital signs and observing his lethargy, which would have to suffice as the baseline for her. I gathered a few guts, took a deep breath, and asked if she could tell roughly how long we had with him. She said she thought about six months, which was considerably longer than I had expected.

I questioned the status of my remaining emotional marbles and Jeffrey's desire to stay... or go. I also theorized that maybe Mary didn't want her speculation to sound too gloomy on the first visit and that maybe she knew six months was probably stretching it. She assured me Jeffrey would remain comfortable to the end, the most welcomed words I'd heard in a long time. I felt an instant rapport with Mary and hoped she would be the nurse assigned to Jeffrey's care, adding to our ever-expanding collection of earth angels (and nurses named Mary!).

Soon after the first hospice group left, two more staff members arrived and stayed another couple of hours for the tedious paperwork duties. While one asked questions, the other glanced at what she presumed was the couch and asked only if she could fold the massive mound of clothes, clean at one time, anyway, and very likely held over from the preacher's visit. Another angel! Or maybe she was just trying to make an indentation for sitting down. I had enough sense to give her permission and wondered if she'd like to vacuum.

I crawled into bed that night fully impacted by the five hours with hospice that day. *Hospice*... whose admirable and much-appreciated purpose was to make dying at home a comfortable, peaceful, and dignified experience for all involved in the process.

The notion that we were, indeed, preparing for the final stages of this assignment, packed on top of unimaginable, indescribable fatigue and anxiety over what would come next, signaled the floodgates to part.

And the tears flowed. And flowed.

Fifty-nine

The entire next day was governed by at least one full moon.
Nellie and the phone both decided to go wacky on us with
bizarre behavior, joining in the madness of the entire fam-
ily and anyone who inhaled. I found a scrap of paper on which
Matthew had written, *Sometimes life sucks, and sometimes it don't.*
An astute observation... and an understatement.

The yard guy came down from mowing the top of the mountain and around the old cemetery after being stung on the leg by
a bee. I got some of the liquid cure-all herbs I'd used for Jeffrey's
earlier massages and offered the bottle to him; thank goodness
Mom was here to play nurse for him. He said, "Boy, gonna have
tuh git me some uh-this." I smiled faintly and said, "Oh, good—
does it work?" And he smiled back and and said, "No."

Our looniness was contagious... no question.

Matthew's latest Jeffrey questions offered me an opportunity to elaborate about hospice and its new role in our lives, that
keeping Jeffrey as comfortable as possible was now our focus and
would enable him to stay with all of us, with relative ease, until
the end. Hospice would see to it.

Matthew continued to express serious concern about how we
would notify him if something happened during the school day,
so I assured him we wouldn't have him and Katie paged on the
intercom as he'd feared (leading him to dread announcements).
I told him we would go directly to their classrooms to get them.
He beamed with relief and left the room, only to return with another glum face minutes later with, "Now I'll just have to worry
every time the door opens." Poor child.

Mary, officially assigned as Jeffrey's hospice nurse, phoned to say that the prescription she had ordered for Jeffrey was ready and had to be picked up that day. Randy left for the medical wonder drug that would ease Jeffrey's days until our services as his earth family were no longer requested. When he returned, I ripped open the package and read the label of the golden syrup. *Morphine.* I was grateful to have something for Jeffrey's comfort—whatever it took—but administer morphine to our child? Our baby?

This assignment wasn't getting any easier.

The boys went to their usual Friday night football game, while Katie went with Mom on some errands. At the grocery store, Katie discovered a drawing for a Beanie Baby, so while Mom shopped, Katie kept herself busy with the registration slips at the display. She confidently informed Mom, "I just know I'll win, 'cause I filled out all the slips!"

Such confidence and spirit and joy. Such love of life and Beanie Babies and all that an 8-year old should be enjoying.

I prayed at least some of it would remain intact after SMA's round of destruction was complete.

Sixty

A third of October slipped by. Several nights near the beginning of the month had been relatively uneventful, but then Jeffrey began whimpering at night when he stirred. I'd tried feeding him several times during the periods of restlessness, but all he wanted to do was cuddle. So we did.

When he awoke the morning of the 11th, he was fairly clammy; the oxygenator tubing had slipped from its requisite position during my catnap. Feeling a surge of incompetence, I took him downstairs, repositioned the tubing, and watched with wonder and relief as he perked up instantaneously.

He hadn't nursed much even by midmorning, but as he didn't act hungry, I tried not to over-interpret it. My new emotional struggle, added to the ever-present fear that he would choke or aspirate and I couldn't help him, was that he would want to suck but lack the muscles to do so. Then what? Temporarily, anyway, that concern was eventually eased when he nursed before dozing again.

By now Jeffrey was approaching five months of age, and he was beginning to delight himself and us with normal baby discoveries, like his hands. He had spied them earlier, but he began taking them (favoring his left) to his mouth and nibbling on them. I remembered watching with glee the same discoveries by Matthew and Katie; now, the fact that Jeffrey could move his arm at all was enough to spark pride and joy.

Music ignited his smile. He loved Mom's original lullabies for him, and he tolerated even my warbled versions of 'Old Mac-Donald' and 'Wheels on the Bus.' I had long stopped dwelling on the likelihood that he would never sing them with me, or to me.

Jeffrey had been sleeping more since the Asheville adventure, and, even in sleep, his eyes were often left half-opened, a quirk I'd noticed on occasion since his birth. I didn't know if it might be a typical SMA idiosyncrasy or not, but as long as it didn't worsen and/or seem to pose complications, I tried to ignore it as much as possible. In the afternoon, I noticed the dark circles under his eyes and shuddered to think what my own looked like.

The bonus on October 11 was a surprise visit from Ruthie, my unflappable assistant who had worked with me during a few special-needs summer camps and in the classroom my last year at Brockman School. 'Grandma Fay' was enthralled with Jeffrey, and he graced his vibrant, dark-skinned adoptive grandma with his glorious grin. Ruthie's presence, laugh, and humor, even if only a small dose with her brief visit, provided me with enough spark to finish the day.

And at the end of the day, I realized that things had been calm... very calm.

Almost eerily so.

Sixty-one

We were treated on October 12 to a showstopper back-to-myself smile from Jeffrey—a miracle and cause for celebration! It was amazing to witness his recuperation far away from the white coats and medical technology. The eerie calm from the previous night lingered, and, deciding to take advantage of whatever calm we could get, I actually experienced peace and contentment for a change.

Katie, on the other hand, had a particularly rough time grappling with the idea of not having Jeffrey around. When he was obviously feeling terrific, it was especially hard to grasp the threat of losing him. It was also easier—even for just a few minutes—to drift back into Pretend Land and convince ourselves we were simply bystanders in someone else's nightmare. We welcomed any and all respites from the truth we could muster.

Katie asked Jeffrey at one point in the day if he was going to be an angel. He zeroed in on her chocolate brown eyes with his own and beamed at her with his secret.

While I sometimes wondered if God talked to me in response to my questions, I had no doubts He must be talking to Jeffrey.

Sixty-two

Over the next few days, life seemed almost simple. Jeffrey enjoyed scoping out his hands and holding his paci with the top of his hand before pushing it back into his mouth. It was a new accomplishment, *normal*, and great fun to watch!

Another major event occurred—I took a shower. I had been taking Jeffrey everywhere (everywhere defined as rare flights to the bathroom and even the computer), but it had become increasingly difficult. He was beginning to reach distress levels in less time without the blow-by oxygen, so I didn't stray far. A shower was a luxury.

Mom's birthday was the 16th; her gift from us was persuading her to stay home (at the lodge) instead of coming over to help. She came to help later, anyway.

I began to feel increased confidence that the end for Jeffrey would be peaceful, but the prayers continued for the order. I had no idea when it would end, but there was no rush as long as Jeffrey felt so good. It was wonderful to enjoy him in an almost-normal baby environment!

On October 18, Jeffrey turned five months old, and we celebrated with drizzly, dreary weather. Matthew and Katie acted like humans toward each other, and Randy and Jeffrey watched football on TV while I attempted unsuccessfully to take a nap in a horizontal position.

Jeffrey's diaper again revealed something orange and crusty, but as Paul still had no clues and Jeffrey still didn't seem bothered, I decided it still didn't warrant extra concern from me. He and I spent a restless night in the Jeffrey chair, as he whimpered quietly for hours. The next morning, he was still restless but was beginning to take to his mouth whatever he could get. I thought he might be teething—another normal baby event. Was it possible? As his whimpering continued, I gave him some grape Tylenol, which he guzzled down happily, and he talked to Nana during her daily visit more than ever, expressing pure admiration for the pictures (of himself) she showed him.

That night, Jeffrey and I actually slept in bed for three hours, enabling my poor sausage feet to ponder shriveling. We were back in the Jeffrey chair by 3am for a very few hours, when Katie began squawking loudly that she looked like the Addams family (her hair *was* a fright), her socks didn't fit, her shoes wouldn't go on, and Nellie was in her way. Etc., etc., etc. She would be perfect in her role as a robber in her reading group's play later in the day, provided her character indulged in his life of crime as a grouch. At least she had already found her robber outfit—jeans and a bandana. "WHEW! I'm wearing other clothes and *taking* my jeans and shirt so I won't be humiliated all day." You go, girl.

One obvious new development was the ease and speed with which Jeffrey could zip from the okay end of the spectrum all the way to the not okay extreme. One minute he appeared 'fine,' the next I was frantically suctioning him to provide immediate relief. During one nursing and later, another, his nostrils flared and milk dribbled out of his nose. I felt sure—I thought—that we were winding down, but I wasn't sure how fast or even how to react. Functional numbness began easing back.

October 21 signaled two weeks since the trip to Asheville, and Jeffrey had done quite well in general. The toll of the overall journey thus far continued, however, and we relished every positive event. Katie beamed with pride when she earned a spot in the I-Can-Manage-Myself club at school for getting her 'aluminum sentences' done, but her greatest joy stemmed from the enormous Jeffrey smiles whenever she doted on him. He loved the Beanie Baby monkey she shared enthusiastically with him, but not nearly as much as he obviously loved her.

I knew that somehow we would all be more adept at handling challenges after this, but I wondered how Matthew and Katie, so young and otherwise unfamiliar with life's hard knocks, would fare without their baby brother. How would any of us fare? This was more than a hard knock.

It was an avalanche.

Sixty-three

The arrival of October 22 began with the mysterious appearance on our front porch of the biggest cabbage we'd ever seen. We snatched it up, considering it a sign of someone's generosity or sense of humor, if nothing else.

I tried to bathe Jeffrey on his new bath sponge, thinking he would feel refreshed after a bath, but he became too distressed. Back to dinky sponge baths for both of us. It was a good thing our social calendar was empty.

Mary came in the afternoon to check Jeffrey's vital signs. He seemed more agitated during the exam and turned a dusky color, which Mary explained was air hunger, the inability of the decreased oxygen supply to reach non-vital parts of the body like skin.

The air hunger served as notice that time had come for the initial dose of morphine. Mary measured the morphine into the syringe and eased it into Jeffrey's mouth, squirting gently. And then she handed the syringe to me to empty out the syringe. Sure enough, within seconds, he pinked up before settling down into a comfortable sleep.

Giving Jeffrey morphine left me somewhat limp, but I did feel a sense of calm and gratitude that it had worked so quickly. My fear of Jeffrey's losing his swallowing ability was diluted sufficiently by Mary's explanation that his body would be close to shutting down at that point. Thank goodness.

Fifteen minutes after Mary left, Jeffrey woke up smiling. I renewed my determination to do whatever it took to keep him happy and comfortable for however long we had with him.

Whatever it took. More prayers.

Dad found a monstrous praying mantis on the road in front of our house when he came over later in the day. We had requested all the prayer assistance we could muster and didn't question the source. I figured God must have sent a praying insect as His gift of comical rejuvenation to us.

Katie was thrilled and rushed inside to find a picture of a praying mantis in her wildlife book. She managed to procure for our confiscated green guy a potential mate from the book and howled, "Look—he's trying to get out to his true love!" I had no doubt he was, indeed, attempting to get out, damsel or not.

Not missing a beat, she then looked up praying mantis on the Internet and hollered, "THEY HAVE THEIR OWN WEB SITE!!!" Those mantises, praying or otherwise, turned out to be a rock group, which made the whole thing even more ridiculous, as under a rock was probably where ours would have preferred hiding at that moment. We relished the absurdity and momentary interruption from reality.

Jeffrey went back to sleep after about an hour of feeling good and slept over five hours before I picked him up just to hold him… as if I weren't already doing that virtually all the time.

The insurance person at Dr. Cade's office called to report that Medicaid had sent them an ugly letter, claiming they didn't know Jeffrey was also covered by another insurance company and demanding a refund for all they had sent on Jeffrey's behalf ($79, which might as well have been $79,000). We were to send the doctor full payment immediately. Sure thing—hop in line.

Paul came to help Randy replace the posts barely holding the house together, and neighbors brought over a cake. Dad arrived under the guise of checking on the posts, but as it was dark, I felt certain he was checking on Jeffrey. He worried that Jeffrey was suffering, although Mom tried to convince him that he wasn't.

If I was certain, or almost certain, of only one thing, it was that Jeffrey had never endured pain from the SMA itself, and wouldn't, either, with Mary and morphine on our side.

After wrapping up work on the posts, Randy and Matthew headed up the stairs at 8:00 that evening to watch the World Series, and I never saw either of them again that night. I realized I had a splitting headache and that my teeth were sore. I guessed I could add 'Grinding teeth' to my resume for application to the rubber room.

After another brief round of snoozing, Jeffrey opened his eyes, drowsy but smiling some. He hadn't wanted to nurse or take his paci all day, and after an hour, he drifted back to sleep.

At 1am, I went upstairs with our tiny slumbering prince and his paraphernalia to attempt sleeping in bed. Randy was fast asleep, and Matthew was equally conked out beside him on my side of the bed. Not easily defeated, I took Jeffrey to Matthew's bed, which was covered in Legos. Oops. Then I went to Katie's bed, which was covered in Katie. So with a rare opportunity to sleep once again in a real bed, there was no bed!

Even Goldilocks had eventually found something that worked.

But then, that was a fairy tale.

Sixty-four

October 23—I was still awake in the chair at 3am, with Jeffrey sleeping in my lap, my head pounding, and tears gushing. The image of handing Jeffrey over to a funeral home had stealthily invaded my throbbing head and refused to vacate. It was the most painful image yet—giving him up forever. While I knew in my heart that his spirit would remain with us, it was the fact that he would be out of my arms before long that currently permeated my soul. The agony of that reminder fortified my excruciating head-in-a-vise-with-a-hammer-ache.

At 3:10am, I decided that in order to function in any capacity, sleep was mandatory. I closed my eyes, and one minute later, Jeffrey woke up for a snack before drifting back to sleep. At 4am, I was still reeling from the punishing sledgehammer on my head. I considered the disturbing possibility that it might be permanent.

When Randy woke up, the thermometer outside indicated nineteen degrees, so the heater was fired up in a jiffy. I instantly began thinking about the likely effects of cold weather on Jeffrey and his respiratory system and quickly deemed its deadly potential too frightening for further contemplation at the moment. We weren't going anywhere, anyway.

There was no school scheduled for students that day due to teacher conferences and report cards, which Dad volunteered to pick up for us. Somehow, Matthew and Katie had both continued doing amazingly well in school. We were so proud of them and in awe of their accomplishments in the classroom, particularly in the midst of such emotional turbulence.

Jeffrey awoke around 10am quite perky, but within minutes

he was fussing and turning dusky. Acting like a seasoned pro, I inserted the scheduled .6ml of morphine into his mouth, and he relaxed almost before I withdrew the syringe. He fell right back asleep for an hour, after which he nursed a little in a rather dazed state. His eyes opened frequently, but he was most certainly in la-la land. I didn't want to think we would have to rely on sedation for the remainder of his days, but I didn't want him to be uncomfortable, either. What a choice.

At 8:35pm, Jeffrey needed another dose of morphine, and I almost felt envious when he drifted off to sleep, as my head still pounded with unrelenting insistence. Three hours later, I went to bed, placing Jeffrey carefully between Randy and me, grateful for the chance to sleep in bed. Never again would I take sleeping on a real mattress for granted.

Jeffrey awoke at 4:30am, a little gurgly but not in distress. I took him downstairs to the chair, knocking over everything in the path of the oxygenator's tubing, and fed him. Afterwards, he seemed content but almost instantly began whimpering. I readied another syringe with morphine (once a Scout, always a Scout. *Be prepared.*). When I finished reloading the syringe and returned my full attention to him, he was already dozing. His eyes then suddenly popped open, and he was smiling!

Thanks to our participation in this yo-yo game of inconsistent behavior, I felt wackier by the minute and overqualified to join the world of hopeless insanity, especially when recalling my bizarre dream of the previous night. Two women had injected themselves in a suicide attempt and yet maintained their regular order of business—with no sign of any progress in their endeavor—for the entire duration of the dream, which could have lasted five minutes (the amount of time I felt like I had slept) or five hours, the length of time I'd spent in one position in varying degrees of unconsciousness.

Adding to the morning commotion, Katie woke up at 7:20am, allowing her a whopping ten minutes to get ready for school. At least vanity hadn't introduced itself yet. The fact that she and her hair could have qualified for disaster relief didn't faze her.

Thank goodness for small favors.

Sixty-five

Randy and I awoke on October 25, each of us feeling like we'd slept in a vise. Our backs were aching in a big way, and Jeffrey was restless. I took his outfit off in a hopeful attempt to settle him down and see a smile. It worked, until—out of nowhere and without any rational encouragement—my lone brain cell screamed, "INSURANCE!" I realized in horror that I had forgotten to pay the premium for the health insurance. In a slight panic, I hoped Randy remembered where he'd put the bill, and I hoped I remembered where I'd last tossed the checkbook. I was afraid to discover what else I had forgotten and thankful my head was attached in the literal sense, anyway.

The morning followed in fitting fashion. At 8:30am, Jeffrey felt good and was smiling. Four minutes later came a downward spiral—mute cry, frantic eyes, and poor color—so I gave him morphine. Ten minutes later, there was no improvement, so I triple-checked the chart for the total amount I could give within the time frame and gave him more. It took five minutes for the desired result, significantly longer than usual. I also had to suction him, as he was gurgly, and the secretions were more plentiful and thicker than before. Not good.

Two hours later, mid-morning, Jeffrey woke up in semiconsciousness and smiled. He acted like he wanted to nurse, but the milk just trickled out of his mouth. It didn't seem he couldn't suck, though, another sign for which I stayed on full alert. He continued dozing with his eyes at half-mast, while I observed just how long—and thin—he had become.

After a relatively uneventful rest of the day, Jeffrey awoke at 5:35pm in significant distress. I quickly gave him the scheduled serving of morphine, which calmed him down immediately without knocking him out. He then smiled, cooed, and waved his arms for over an hour before drifting off to sleep. At 10:05pm, he awoke in distress again, so I gave him additional morphine.

The irregular breathing pattern, which Mary had identified as Cheyne-Stokes, began forty-five minutes later. More morphine. His breathing became increasingly shallow, and his color was frightening. I asked Katie to get Randy, as it seemed much too close to the end. At that point, we had agonized eight times in thinking the end was nearing. I wondered again how many rehearsals we needed.

Randy joined us, expressing his childhood fear of not being able to breathe, thanks to severe allergies. Now he watched his child struggle in his place, which was tough. Our newest blessing was the morphine.

At 11pm, I looked over the morphine schedule to see when Jeffrey could have the next dose and realized in disbelieving horror that after all my meticulous calculations, it was completely wrong, as I had already changed the clocks back for the end of daylight savings time. I had to refigure hastily, translating the old times into the new times before Jeffrey needed another dose.

I would have been bonkers enough with the chore had I been alert, but my brain was shot, rendering the task one of mass frustration, confusion, and tears. I finally thought I might have figured it out, and Jeffrey and I headed to bed.

Another weird dream floated through my gray matter. I found a big hunk of cheese, with bites out of one end, that had fallen on a concrete floor under what appeared to be a pew or bench.

Would I need my toothbrush in the rubber room?

Sixty-six

Around 1am on the 26th of October, Jeffrey cried out in our bed, so I took him downstairs and got us situated for the day's events. I hoped it wasn't the beginning of a crisis, as with the corrected morphine schedule, his next dose wouldn't come for almost an hour. His color was good, and his eyes possessed a serious concentration, almost as if he were studying my face for his own assignment. It was a familiar gaze, but at first I couldn't place where I had seen it before.

Then I remembered. It was the same expression Duffy had in his eyes after he'd been hit by the car and that Paul had in his eyes after examining Jeffrey... such an eerie, seemingly apparent calm and control of the situation. Of course, Duffy had been in shock, as had Paul, to a considerable degree, so was this It? I watched his breathing, which was steady and relatively strong, and he fell asleep twenty-five minutes later.

After about an hour and a half, Jeffrey woke up and tried to nurse, but he had a tough time sucking, in spite of the effort he was putting into it. I helped as much as I could by squeezing the milk into his mouth. He dozed off again, this time with peaceful, shallow breathing, while I tried to prepare myself for the inevitable. His eyelids parted just slightly, as if he were already in transit.

At 8:05am, Jeffrey was still sleeping and had had no morphine in nine hours. Two hours later, he threw up yellow goop, a new event. Two hours after that, he nursed with relative ease. Every single moment seemed to bring the unexpected. My guard remained steadfastly in place—wobbly, but up.

Mom came to take Katie shopping, and Randy and Matthew

left on errands. While everyone was gone, I decided to make a quick run to the bathroom, gently placing Jeffrey in the cradle to avoid disturbing him any more than necessary. He immediately went into distress, so I gave him morphine.

When he conked out, I gently put him down again. I rushed to the bathroom and back with impressive speed and found he had already returned to a state of distress. I grabbed the syringe for more morphine and upped the oxygen, but his color was still not good. I moved on to the next item on the agenda... suctioning. That helped some, at least for the time being. I figured we were nearing the point when it wouldn't have a noticeable impact.

Matthew asked later in the day what my biggest fear or worry was. At that moment, I could honestly say it was the feeling that the chaos and anguish that had become such a way of life would never end and that I would worry about Jeffrey forever. That was immediately countered, however, by the thought that in reality, this would end before too long and that I wouldn't be nearly as prepared as I claimed to be. However, on still another flip side, I'd thought the end was near about nine times before. Obviously, I had no clue, and it would very probably stay that way.

Jeffrey required suctioning numerous times throughout the day for what looked like milk in his cheeks. Not only did he seem to appreciate the benefits of the suctioning, though, he even smiled. If our little guy was able to find something—anything—to smile about after all he'd been through, then that was the lesson for the rest of us to remember from then on.

At 3:40pm, Jeffrey was still restless, but as there were over two hours until the next scheduled morphine dose, I called Mary for advice. She arrived in twenty minutes and gave Jeffrey .5ml morphine, then waited to check his respiration. I couldn't envision halting the delivery of morphine in times of distress if complications had arisen; thankfully, if there had been side effects, they were too negligible for concern.

Mary told us how much more we could begin giving him each hour if necessary. Sure enough, the extra dose seemed to ease Jeffrey's discomfort quickly, and he nursed quite well before falling asleep for over seven hours. He woke up and nursed again, feeling good. He and I watched the final couple of minutes of the World Series (the Marlins finally won in the twelfth inning), and he ate once more before conking out a little after midnight, again without benefit of morphine or suctioning!

I wondered if it was the calm before the storm.

Sixty-seven

Jeffrey awoke at 4:15am on October 27, a little fussy but comforted with some milk and cuddling for about an hour before nodding off again, and still without recent benefit of morphine or suctioning. I realized with a bit of fascinated disgust just how inflated my legs, feet, and knees had become from sitting in the Jeffrey chair on a semi-permanent basis and dreaded the thought of shoving my pig feet into real shoes.

A neighbor called at 7:10am to check on Jeffrey. At the precise moment of the question, he was actually fine. At the precise moment of Randy's positive report, however, Jeffrey rebutted by plunging promptly into a state of distress, requiring morphine followed immediately by suctioning. Thirty minutes later, additional morphine was needed, and then he fell asleep.

Two and a half hours later, Jeffrey opened his eyes wide and eyeballed me with a rather odd expression. I wondered if he thought I was going to leave him, or maybe we were fast approaching the time when he would leave us. Or maybe he was just eyeballing me with a rather odd expression.

At 4pm, after being awake and feeling good for about an hour, Jeffrey needed more morphine and wanted more music. I obliged first with the morphine, then tried to reach and operate the cassette recorder with my toes, as it was out of my hands' reach. Unfortunately, my former toes had ballooned to the size of Polish sausages and were a bit thick for usefulness.

The tape in the cassette player, consisting of lullabies Mom had composed for Jeffrey, had been playing over and over and over for weeks, and as it was a source of comfort for Jeffrey and soothing for my own nerves, I managed to get it started again with a final boost of determination.

The evening brought with it a bit of cheap entertainment. Katie began crying because she couldn't 'do anything,' then Matthew started because Katie was crying. Then I joined in because they were crying. Randy left for the mountain top with Nellie, who was equally grateful for an escape. Jeffrey slept through the whole thing. Quality family time at its finest.

Matthew continued asking questions, such as what we were going to do with all the medical equipment, and then he said, "I'm worried about how my classmates will react." I knew they'd react with compassion and would respect his needs, whatever they happened to be, but there was no way to convince Matthew. The time would simply have to come for us to discover just how bumpy the next stretch of the journey would be. I thought the waiting would be over soon.

I realized, during the course of the discussion with Matthew, that the one task we wouldn't have to complete was the dismantling of a room for Jeffrey—what a relief! I had always envisioned that to be one of the toughest duties facing parents after a child's death, but we were spared.

Thank you, dear Lord. Again.

Sixty-eight

Not long after midnight on October 28, the day began for Jeffrey with some difficulty nursing. He was happy to cuddle, though, and he loved being massaged with a cool rag, especially on his head, while he listened to Nana's Jeffrey music. We had listened to the tape so many times the past few weeks, it was a miracle it hadn't rebelled by snapping in two. Angels must have been holding it together.

I could probably say the same for me.

At 3:15am, peculiar 'belch' sounds came from Jeffrey three times, providing a flashback to the final death bellow from one of our dogs years before. For the umpteenth time, I wondered if that was how it would end and tried to ready myself mentally and emotionally. Again. At 4:55am, Jeffrey threw up, and his body was hot. Thirty minutes later, the morphine was put to use, enabling him to sleep for almost an hour.

At 9am, which seemed like three days after he'd first awakened that morning, he needed morphine. Forty minutes later, he needed more; afterwards he slept, woke up to nurse, then slept again.

No additional morphine was required for almost four hours. I was getting through the days by measuring in increments of four hours. I had become as dependent on the morphine schedule as I was on the clock in gauging the time and its passage. That's not to say I comprehended time and its passage.

At 6:00 that evening, I wondered if maybe I needed to pack in earnest for the rubber room... or if it was too late. Jeffrey was still asleep, and I could not remember if he'd been awake at all during the day. And if I thought he'd been awake, could it possibly have been the day before I was thinking about? I was getting nuttier by the minute. That was not comforting, as I hadn't had a lot of sense to play with in the beginning. By the end of the day, I was hearing things, mostly music, although I wasn't sure if it was something I'd heard before or something my brain was making up.

I wondered if it mattered.

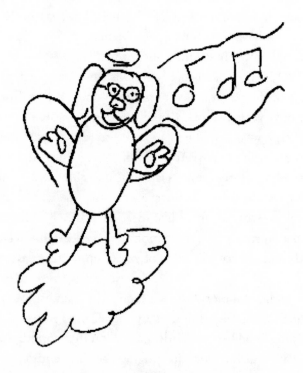

Sixty-nine

October 29—I had fallen asleep in the Jeffrey chair until a little past midnight. Since Jeffrey was sound asleep on my lap, I made a daring attempt to take him and the tubing upstairs to bed with Randy. I could have slept without a moment's hesitation, but I decided I'd better take advantage of whatever spare minutes I might have and tend first to necessities that were often unattainable, like a shower. I then collapsed in bed at 1am, dozing over an hour until Jeffrey needed to move back to the chair.

Four hours later, I gave Jeffrey morphine to ease his distress and expected him to fall asleep. He did... for ten minutes. He awoke with bright eyes and a lot of jabbering, which was always a treat, regardless of the time. Katie popped up out of bed at 6am, got dressed, and read, all on her own.

I wondered if aliens had come during the night.

Mary was scheduled to check Jeffrey that morning. Before her arrival, I observed how bony Jeffrey's head had become and, again, how long and thin he was. And beautiful. His features were simply perfect and, while the cuddly, chubby baby look had vanished, his thinness afforded easy access to his delicate features... just like a fine porcelain doll.

Jeffrey needed more morphine right before Mary's arrival. She examined him and didn't hear much coming out of his right lung, but his left lung seemed clear.

She then quietly informed me that there was medication for depression, which tends to set in about three weeks after the onset of a crisis. Since we had been in full force for a while longer, she said it would be more unusual for us not to be depressed.

Interestingly to me, I hadn't felt depressed in the usual sense for extended periods, although I was most certainly down and extremely exhausted mentally, emotionally, and physically. Spiritually, I believed I was in remarkably good condition.

Mary commented on the slight increase in movement of Jeffrey's arms (maybe I wasn't imagining it after all) and also said she would handle the removal of all the medical equipment when the time came. I didn't balk.

Mom came just as Mary was leaving. As soon as Jeffrey was placed in his spot on her lap, she commented how much he was jabbering to her. Maybe more than ever. I remained curious as to what he had been chattering about the past couple of weeks.

Mom also mentioned that Dad was crushed by the situation we were facing, and that she had tried to assure him our immediate focus was on making Jeffrey comfortable, not on the end.

That was how we had remained upright in our journey so far, tackling each immediate objective/crisis without focusing on the final result per se. Baby steps.

And grown-up prayers.

Seventy

The day was absolutely gorgeous, and Randy almost smiled for the first time in months. He had decided that his contribution for Jeffrey would be a memorial chapel on top of our little mountain, near the site he'd planned for Jeffrey and the old cemetery. He had in mind something small and simple, dependent on natural light and a wood-burning fireplace, and with plenty of windows for easy access to the heavens. It was a perfect idea! I knew it would be a masterpiece, and it would also serve as a terrific mode of therapy for Randy and the rest of us. Sparked by Randy's enthusiasm and appreciative of any positive action for 'later,' I then wondered what else our family could come up with for Jeffrey.

That night, bolstered by the optimism of the day, I made a concerted effort to really *see* Jeffrey before it was too late: long, dark, wavy hair with the Elvis-do on top; long lashes and alert, dark chocolate brown eyes; dimples above each corner of his mouth, creating a killer smile; perfectly-formed ears, lips, hands, feet, and skin; long, hairy fingers and legs, with Randy's eclectic toes; his tiny concave chest; small reddish birthmark on his right eyelid; animated facial expressions; open mouth- and partially open-eyed sleeping; remnants of cradle cap; increased amount of sweating, no matter how cool even his hot-natured mama was; fascination with his hands and waving them daintily.

What he loved: being massaged, with and without lotion; being naked; any attention from Matthew or Katie (Katie placed herself on almost-constant call with the crazy leg game, while Matthew elicited a huge smile with his "Let's talk about mucous" line); my lap and his pillow on it; cuddling; nursing; his Nuk silicone paci; the music Nana composed for him; Papa's sweet 'Jeffrey' voice; 'Old MacDonald' and 'Wheels on the Bus'; Nana's blue brush airplane game; a damp cloth on his forehead; playing in the tub; watching football and baseball games on TV with Randy; peek-a-boo.

What we particularly loved: his neon smile and big, bright, all-knowing eyes, and his sweet and cheery disposition. His grace and bravery. There were numerous endearing nicknames for our little guy—Handsome, Sweet Potato, Sweet Pea, Honey Bunny, Little Man—and he glowed at the sound of them all.

What I wouldn't forget: the smell of oxygen flowing through the tubing and the perpetual checking for necessary adjustment of the tubing; the constant hum of the oxygenator; the ever-ready syringe of morphine and the scribbled morphine schedule notes; a peppermint-y Jeffrey after an herbal/oil massage; his Boynton aerobics pillowcase; the constant check of e-mails for news, information, and/or encouragement from other SMA families; the $!*# suction machine; the Jeffrey chair; Mom's soothing *Dreams for Jeffrey* cassette; the concern, love, and prayers from so many folks.

Standard conversational tidbits from the family that no doubt held a permanent place in my memory: from Randy's, "Is he OK?" "What's the matter?" "He sounds gurgly," to Matthew's, "Did he have a good day?" "How's he been doin' today?" "Did he have a good night?" to Katie's, "YOU JUST NEED SISSY! I'M GONNA MOVE DOZE LEGS, YESSA I AM!" and "You gonna be an angel?"

Without any doubt, the answer in Jeffrey's dazzling smile: *Yessa, I am.*

Seventy-one

After my mental inventory of a few Jeffrey memories, I fed him, then headed upstairs to bed, where I gently propped Jeffrey on pillows between Randy and me. I had just settled down and begun dozing when Randy woke me that Jeffrey needed suctioning. Back downstairs we went, my back in spasms. At 1:40am, he needed morphine. Five minutes later, he needed more.

October 30 continued with an apparent decrease in sucking and swallowing abilities. I began squirting milk into Jeffrey's mouth but immediately needed to suction it out. He seemed to be feeling quite comfortable, though, without an overabundance of morphine.

I noticed what looked suspiciously like more hair on the back of the chair than on my head; I would be bald before too many more days. There was no mercy in this game where stress ruled.

Jaymie e-mailed about a gown she was making for Jeffrey's send-off. It was a replica of an antique Victorian day gown she had seen, and she added that he would look like the angel he was. I said a prayer of thanks for her compassion and genuine empathy and for thinking of such a special contribution, and for Paul's support, medical-wise, brother-wise, and otherwise. I thanked God for keeping my parents upright and for the prayers from those in the family who were not nearby.

There was a prayer of thanks for all the countless others who had intervened somehow on Jeffrey's and our behalf in an effort to smooth the road on this part of our journey. Another prayer for the other families dealing with this nightmare—those I knew about, those joining the SMA family in the future, and the many,

many more who would remain anonymous for one reason or another. There was a prayer of gratitude for the good health of Matthew and Katie and even one of hope for their children's good health. I thanked God for enabling Randy and me to remain relatively sturdy throughout this assignment and supportive of each other. Finally, there was a heavy-duty prayer of thanks for our intensifying faith in God. Despite my occasional accusations to the contrary, He had never strayed from us.

I trusted there was no prayer limit, as they flowed, like my tears, without an end in sight.

Seventy-two

October 31—the day of spooks and frights, as if we needed more of either. I dreamed during a quick catnap that
I had ridden to the park on my bike with Katie perched
behind me. When we arrived, we saw nothing but endless rows
of chairs, Beanie Babies filling all the seats on the front row. In
this park, you just sat... like a Beanie Baby.

But in this real world of ours, there was no such thing as just
sitting. At 6:25am, I gave Jeffrey a dose of breakfast morphine.
His heart was pounding, and he was having trouble swallowing.
He required immediate suctioning farther down his throat than
usual, causing me to wonder how much morphine he actually
absorbed. Five minutes later, I gave him more morphine, and
fifteen minutes later, a little more. Five minutes after that, still
more, until he finally settled down. Amid this excitement, Katie
began squawking that she couldn't get dressed with the TV on,
and within minutes, she had mastered "Shut up!" We would all
need therapy.

Matthew donned his new black jeans and new sweatshirt,
courtesy of Nana and Papa. He was quite proud of his new outfit
and quietly said, "I've always wanted black jeans." First I'd heard
of it, but I kept my mouth closed in the likely event that he had
mentioned something about it in a previous life.

After everyone had left for school, I dissolved into tears. My
heart and head had been in perpetual conflict for almost three
and a half months, and even though I was pretty convincing to
myself that we could let Jeffrey go when it was time, the morning's mini-morphine marathon left no doubt in what was left of
my mind that it would be a miserable acknowledgment.

My fear of Jeffrey's choking and my not being able to save him intensified immensely, and the tears flowed until right before Randy returned from morning carpool. He brought back with him a book sent by Debbie, the school counselor angel—Max Lucado's *A Gentle Thunder*, which I managed to finish by noon.

I had already read some of Dr. James Dobson's *When God Doesn't Make Sense*, and I was eager to finish it some day. Both books recounted plentiful examples of hardships endured by seemingly decent, 'undeserving' folks from Biblical times to the present and countless examples of God's grace and love.

Lucado's premise in *A Gentle Thunder* is that God does whatever is necessary to capture our attention in His quest to bring all of us back Home safely. I agreed that our assignment had served as a wake-up call for us, and I tried to reconsider our Jeffrey journey as an opportunity for a better us—not better than everyone else, but better than the old us, which I had sincerely thought was pretty good. We were now refreshingly more attuned to what is really important during our time here.

Without question, we were relying more heavily on prayer with our realization from the beginning that we simply couldn't proceed on this journey alone. The prayers were increasingly tilted more towards sincere gratitude for what we already had as opposed to requests for what we didn't.

I assured myself that God must have thought we all held great potential for something in order for Him to have placed us here in the first place, not to mention the responsibility and privilege of caring for Jeffrey. Thanks to the thrust of our family into a crisis situation, perhaps we were able to see some of the potential God knew we had. It was a consoling thought at the time; I hoped it lingered.

Jeffrey needed morphine at 12:25pm and again ten minutes later. The mail arrived, and in it was a letter from SSI that our application for benefits for Jeffrey had been denied. *See attached,* it read. The attachment may as well have been in Chinese, as it made no sense to me, but in essence, they seemed to think we made too much money. Hmmm… Randy had lost his job, I certainly wasn't employed, gainfully-speaking, and our primary income was now the fledgling carpet-cleaning business, which could hardly qualify as a reliable job yet. Yep, too much money for sure.

I somehow indulged in a quick shower and shaved parts of my legs, which Katie thought worthy of broadcast on the evening news. Randy and Matthew left for their football night out. As soon as they closed the door, I began my Friday-night prayers that nothing too eventful would happen while they were gone.

Left party-less and stuck with the chairbound duo for the evening, Katie resorted to a magic show on TV. When the wives of the magicians came out to help them with illusional 'life-endangering' stunts, Katie commented, "I know why they use their wives… 'cause no one else'll do it." Wise child.

Surprisingly, the evening was uneventful.

Not surprisingly, the night would more than make up for it.

Seventy-three

The month of November began its business less than three hours into the first day with a substantial dose of morphine for Jeffrey. I also noticed that even under a blanket, his left leg was cooler than the rest of his body. As is common with SMA babies, his body's thermostat didn't function efficiently, but at least that was expected.

At 3am, Jeffrey nursed a little. His sucking and swallowing muscles had weakened more, but as he seemed satisfied enough, I tried not to dwell on it and settled down to snooze with him in the chair in anticipation of whatever crises loomed ahead.

Twenty minutes later, the house became quiet... unnaturally quiet, with the exception of Katie's snoring hailing from the couch across from the Jeffrey chair. There was also no light anywhere, from either the night lights scattered throughout the house or power lights from any piece of equipment.

The power was out!

The oxygenator began beeping the alert, and I started calling for Randy, trying carefully to do so without waking up and scaring Katie or Jeffrey. With his ears stopped up from allergies and a serious need for deep sleep, though, Randy couldn't have heard a train crashing through the wall.

Nevertheless, I continued calling for a few minutes, failing to rouse him. Katie heard me, though, and, as I'd expected, was frantic. She was also still mostly asleep, so the pitch-black room put a double whammy on her capacity to become oriented. Matthew heard me not long after, and then he heard the beeping of the machine. Thinking it was the smoke alarm and that we were on fire, he began sliding down the stairs, bonking his head on the landing.

Randy eventually caught on that he was missing out on some serious excitement, so he staggered down the stairs and fumbled around for a flashlight and candles, managing to get enough light to fiddle with the portable oxygen tank, which we'd never used. It was eventually hooked up for service, just as I glanced in the faint flickering of light at Jeffrey's face. He looked way too much like he had in Asheville after he fell into respiratory arrest.

Oh, God!!!

He was limp and not breathing, and what little I could see of his color was simply draining away. Draining... draining. Then his eyes rolled back, as I frantically patted, pounded, and prayed, COME ON, SWEETIE! COME ON, JEFFREY! Surely this wasn't the way we were ending this journey... or maybe God hadn't wanted us to watch him leave. Well, it was too late! I'd already seen him, and I wasn't about to let him go. Not yet.

After a few long minutes of desperate prodding, I had Matthew hold the oxygen tubing close to his nose (Jeffrey's, not his own, although he probably could have used some himself). It was occasionally misdirected into Jeffrey's nose, but the intentions were honest.

I gave Jeffrey more morphine and suctioned like crazy a little ways down his throat. I didn't appreciate or even comprehend at that time that the battery on the suction machine was functioning.

Katie did her best to hold the flashlight so we could see what we were doing, but her jittery hands waved the light wildly in all directions but the one we needed. Meanwhile, Randy checked the breakers and called the electric company to get us hooked back up as soon as possible, though our earlier placement on the emergency medical needs list would take care of that, anyway. He was informed by the representative that the entire station was out of power.

Jeffrey had begun breathing again, and my mind frantically

grasped for any purpose for that harrowing experience. I wondered if the end wasn't going to be peaceful, after all, and if perhaps God had just tried to spare us by enveloping us in darkness. We were all there, as we'd prayed, but hadn't we also prayed for a calm departure for Jeffrey?

DEAR GOD, HELP US!!!

At least daylight wasn't too many hours away. I flashed back a few years to Hurricane Hugo's vengeance in Columbia, South Carolina. Three-year old Matthew, wearing Randy's old football helmet for protection, slept soundly in the hall closet, month-old Katie snoozing next to him in his play orange football helmet. Randy and I prayed and huddled over them for hours. The entire night was one of sheer terror; we could only imagine what havoc was being wreaked upon us with the thunderous racket in the pitch black outside. When daylight finally arrived upon completion of Hugo's destructive fury, there was a surreal stillness amid the massive upheaval and the most incredibly magnificent, crystalline blue sky imaginable.

I wondered if we would experience that same calm when we inventoried what the wrath of SMA had left in its wake.

Seventy-four

At 3:35am, still in the dark without power, Jeffrey needed more morphine, and Katie headed to the bathroom, promptly knocking over the portable oxygen tank in her path and further frazzling all nerves. The scene was beginning to resemble slapstick comedy, although no one was laughing.

At 4:20am, our prayers were answered with the return of power, courtesy of the electric company. Three hours later, Jeffrey was on his fourth dose of morphine, after which he needed more no-nonsense suctioning. The suction machine battery had become too weak to be of service, at which time I realized how fortunate (blessed) we had been with its cooperation not long before. I thanked God for power—the electric company's and His—and, once again, for the fact that He was in control of this ordeal and not any of us mere mortals.

The day was almost painfully sunny, just as it had been after Hurricane Hugo's visit. Jeffrey seemed especially tired of the commotion, and no one blamed him. The pervasive thought was how much longer he could or would muster the effort to stick around.

A futile attempt at normalcy returned. Randy vacuumed, while Nellie, canine nerves shot into oblivion along with the rest of the family's, promptly threw up right behind him.

At 8:50am, I tried dropping milk into Jeffrey's mouth. He was having increased difficulty sucking and swallowing, and any amount of milk had to be suctioned out. He needed morphine, and since the dose would have to suffice for another two hours, I called Mary to see what we could do if he needed more before then. She offered to come over, but I assured her we were doing okay… for the moment. I really wanted us to be able to do this ourselves if at all possible, surmising that since we had come this far, anything was possible.

Jeffrey had somehow managed to look noticeably thinner than just days before, and his outfits swallowed him. I had no idea how much or how little he weighed, nor did I want to know.

Dad popped over unexpectedly, cleaned out some dead flies in a ceiling light, and left. I figured it was too tough for him to see Jeffrey, and yet he couldn't bear not to see him before his escape, either.

At 11:10am, I squirted more milk into Jeffrey's mouth with a dropper; fifteen minutes later, the milk in the dropper had been replaced with morphine. Matthew's simultaneous announcement of a stomach ache, one side effect of life as we'd come to know it, was hardly a surprise.

At noon, I rushed to the bathroom with Jeffrey in tow, then rushed him back for more morphine. I tried dropping milk into his mouth, first from the dropper, and then straight from my nipple, and then onto the paci, which seemed the most soothing to him. He sucked a little before falling asleep. By that time, I felt somewhat relaxed while he slept; I knew he wasn't in distress then, and I also knew that even if he were to stop breathing during sleep, it would surely be a peaceful departure. Surely.

After the harried events of the night and observations of his rapidly decreasing abilities to suck and swallow, I asked God to take Jeffrey if it was His will to do so. I didn't dare presume I knew more than God, although it seemed questionable to me at times. I figured we were all about as ready as we'd ever be to let go of our little guy, and I didn't know how much more I could handle, worrying about Jeffrey and possible emergency scenarios.

Rejuvenated somewhat shortly after my plea to God, I decided, once again, that we could—and would—handle whatever

He doled out. For however long it took. He had not let us down in this journey.

We wouldn't let Him down, either.

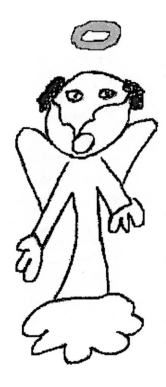

Seventy-five

Toby, who had worked steadily on the Jeffrey road in his quest to finish in time, came over to continue. Even without children of his own, he understood the importance of his contribution to this journey. Once Toby was underway, and as the day had ooched forward without further calamity, Randy and Matthew made a quick escape for some necessary errands.

Mom dropped in during a brief but lively thunderstorm, during which Katie panicked about a possible lightning strike to the television antenna. She rushed upstairs to disconnect the antenna from the TV and to unplug the TV, then went into greater panic when she couldn't get the antenna out. Mom calmly unscrewed it for her, and Katie returned to her bouncy self.

Forget therapy intervention; we were headed straight for a family-size padded cell.

Mom offered to watch Jeffrey while I walked up the new road, but I didn't want to leave him. Besides, I'd see the road soon enough.

At 5:45pm, Jeffrey was on his fourth dose of morphine in two hours. He hadn't smiled all day (who *had*), then I realized there had been only a bare hint of a smile the past two days. I worried that he was unhappy and/or uncomfortable but quickly altered my thinking to assume he was merely focusing on his upcoming transition. Surely it wouldn't be much longer.

At 6:45pm, Jeffrey received a dose of morphine. Less than an hour later, another dose was in order. Randy said he (himself) felt hot to the core, another of the myriad responses to stress in our collection. At 10:05pm, additional morphine resulted in less effect, and we began to assume—hope—that the end was nearing.

It was not an easy thought, nor would it be an easy acceptance when it did come, but we all loved Jeffrey enough to want it to be over for his sake. He had been a tiny warrior long enough.

At 11:35pm, morphine again.

Before bedtime (for the others) on what was still just the first day of a month that had seemed an eternity, Randy switched the baby monitor parts so that I could simply talk to him from the chair in case of another emergency.

It was a great idea, until I realized after he was in bed that he would be hearing the racket of the suctioning machine and the unsettling suctioning process itself for the requisite umpteen times during the night. There would be no sleep for him, either, as if he'd managed any quality sleep lately. I tried to keep things as quiet otherwise as possible and realized again that even when Mom's Jeffrey tape ended its round, I was still hearing the music. I had mastered the art of self-relaxation.

Or else, I was officially crazy.

Was my room ready?

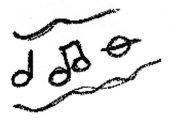

Seventy-six

At midnight, bumping us finally to November 2, my study of the morphine chart indicated that Jeffrey had had only .4cc in the past two hours, which, after the previous day's demands, was barely worth noting. Five minutes later, however, he needed another dose. I tried squirting milk into his mouth, but it didn't work. I then tried water, hoping that if nothing else, it would help keep his mouth from becoming uncomfortably dry.

Forty-five minutes later, Jeffrey received more morphine, along with a soothing massage with lotion on his legs and a cool rag on his forehead. His breathing, erratic and sometimes alarmingly shallow, kept my frazzled body, brain, and soul on call. By 3:15am, he had had four more doses; at 8am, he awoke alert!

He dozed while I was on the phone and nursed with amazing ease an hour later, once again playing the yo-yo game, the rules of which I still hadn't figured out. In less than an hour, before I could finish adjusting emotional gears again, he needed suctioning and more morphine, and twenty minutes later, he simply didn't look good. If God's goal in this journey was to drive me insane, He had succeeded... long ago.

Over the course of the afternoon and evening, Jeffrey required several rounds of morphine to calm his episodes of respiratory distress. In the midst, I received an e-mail from a mom whose six-year old son had received a trach at three months, and she wondered if a trach might be an option for Jeffrey. *SIX YEARS?* I couldn't fathom the torture of enduring SMA—this form of it, anyway—for years. I was sick of the suction machine, sick of the oxygenator tubing, sick of morphine and watching the clock and figuring out dosages and times. More than anything, though, I was exhausted from worrying about Jeffrey and wondering if I had any clue as to what I was doing or if we had done enough.

"God doesn't give us more than we can handle" came to what was left of my senses.

I wondered if He had ever heard that.

Seventy-seven

The third day of November began early with too many morphine doses, suctioning, and a dream that I'd put a chicken in the oven but couldn't tell later if it had been baked or not. Perhaps I'd chugged a bit of the morphine myself... or should have. At 3:30am, Jeffrey had almost reached his morphine allotment for the four-hour period and would be allowed only an insignificant amount for two more hours.

Each minute seemed like infinity.

At 7:30am, I spied red blotches on Jeffrey's neck, behind his left ear, and underneath his chin. I had no clue as to what that might indicate (was there a rash with impending death?) but kept a watch on it. At 8am, he needed morphine. Ten minutes later, the mysterious blotches had disappeared, but he needed deeper suctioning. I began praying—begging—for God to take him before I was carted off.

Jaymie reported that Jeffrey's going-away gown should arrive by 10:30 that morning. I planned to take some pictures of Jeffrey in it, as there would be no pictures later. I knew the gown would be gorgeous. Jaymie had plenty of talent to match the demands she placed on herself to produce nothing less than top quality. She had also made a pillow to accompany him or to leave here. She had thought of it all.

By midmorning, Mom came over, then Dad, then Randy returned from his business. The gown arrived, and it was even more exquisite than I had envisioned. Jaymie wrote that making it had been a bittersweet experience, that she still clung to the remote glimmer of a possibility that it wouldn't be needed, but, she repeated, Jeffrey would look like the angel that he was.

At noon, Jeffrey needed morphine. An hour later, he needed morphine again and suctioning, and a monumental turning point occurred: he clamped his lips shut for both the morphine and suctioning, pleading with his dark chocolate eyes for permission to be excused. That signaled the absolute end of my composure, as he had just provided proof enough that he was ready to exit this madness. I managed to get two more morphine doses into his mouth during the afternoon despite his lack of cooperation, but the thought that he was wanting out was simply unbearable.

This assignment would not be over a moment too soon.

Seventy-eight

Katie arrived home from school and spied the gown immediately. With visions of her American Girl dolls upstairs, she squealed, "Oh! What's this for?"

I was going to have to answer. Her enthusiasm took a nose dive upon hearing the carefully-worded explanation of why Jaymie had made it. Her desire to keep it only increased when I finished fumbling for words, as if refusing to relinquish it would keep Jeffrey here.

DO YOU SEE THIS, GOD? DO YOU SEE WHAT'S HAPPENING HERE? HELP ME! I heard no answer from Him, only the familiar sound of sobbing from Katie and me.

The day, which had started out sunny, had changed to one of gloom and rain with possible snow showers. As had often been the case, the weather mirrored the atmosphere inside. After doling out more morphine and repeated suctioning, anger began pouring out; I suddenly felt particularly cheated having to deal with Jeffrey as a nurse more than as a mama. *WHAT KIND OF GOD ARE YOU TO GIVE A LOVING FAMILY A BABY—AND THEN TAKE HIM AWAY???* Like the rest of the family, I was running on fumes in every capacity of my existence.

Randy and I took the opportunity to discuss in greater detail with Matthew and Katie the plan for contacting them should something happen while they were in school. They both feared the intercom and the opening of the classroom door, so I told them with a halfhearted remnant of humor that we'd just knock on the window. Matthew replied incredulously, "Really—you're gonna knock on the window?" The horror of sheer embarrassment at that prospect overrode his sense of worry about Jeffrey, at least temporarily.

Meanwhile, Katie burst into a marathon bawling session, and not until we diffused it with discussions of the after-Jeffrey's-safe plans of fixing up the cemetery and planting lots of flowers did she calm down enough to offer her own suggestions, such as painting wooden angels taken from her drawings. It would be a beautiful tribute to our very special little guy. That... and therapy for those of us left behind.

After Katie finally conked out, I took a deep breath and apologized, through profuse tears, to God. I told Him we understood He knew what He was doing, and even though we were *in* His plan, we were basically outsiders with respect *to* His plan. We were trying diligently to convince ourselves that since there were blessings in this assignment, we could and would fulfill our Jeffrey responsibilities for as long as the assignment lasted. I asked that He continue to stay right beside us until He was ready to take Jeffrey back. I knew He would.

From 7:40pm to 10:05pm, there were four doses of morphine, and I had to suction even with the paci just dampened with water. Jeffrey's swallowing muscles were now gone, and his sucking muscles weren't far behind. I prayed, trusting God would allow his breathing muscles to stop... soon.

There would be no pictures of Jeffrey in his going-away gown.

Seventy-nine

November 4 arrived in what had become typical fashion. Suctioning and morphine were on tap from early morning, and by 6:50am, Jeffrey had had six doses of morphine. There was a bit of snow on the deck, and I realized it was our niece Bethany's ninth birthday. I could handle Jeffrey's acquisition of angel wings on this day, with a cheerfully optimistic explanation for Bethany (he chose a great day!), but I hadn't wanted the funeral on her birthday. She felt as close to Jeffrey as possible from her own home two hours away, and I had not wanted a birthday reminder for her to be a casket with her baby cousin in it. We were safe on that one. Thank You.

After Matthew and Katie departed for school, Randy left on an all-day carpet cleaning mission, which meant I would be left with the clock for an eternity. Mom came over to help as she had done over the previous weeks, so I handed Jeffrey to her and zoomed toward the bathroom, deciding en route to clean the suctioning tank and tubing first. Before I finished rushing through the task, Mom said he needed suctioning again. She was right. The bathroom would have to wait. Again.

I gave Jeffrey five doses of morphine from 11am to 1:55pm, using the latest schedule of increased morphine approved by Mary. In the early afternoon, Jaymie and Bethany drove up unexpectedly. When I saw who it was, I asked Mom to go out and prepare them both, especially Bethany, for the virtually non-stop suctioning and morphine routine. Bethany had wanted to come (no school for her, thanks to Election Day, which was news to me), but when she saw Jeffrey and the cruel toll of SMA on his frail body, she retreated for the safety and solitude of the computer in another room.

2:35pm—morphine time. Katie came home from school and sat a little while with Bethany, whom she adored. I never learned what they said to each other. Maybe nothing.

4:05pm—another dose of morphine. The counselors from school arrived with a huge feast of roast beef, vegetables, salad, desserts, and drinks, and then they presented us with a meal plan for the next few weeks and generous grocery coupons and cash. We were all overcome with a plethora of emotions, particularly gratitude, as well as the knowledge of why they were taking such good care of us.

5:00pm—morphine

5:30pm—more morphine

Randy took Katie to Brownies that night and headed back home to wait for the meeting to end. I prayed they would both return home before Jeffrey's earthly departure, as he seemed to be winding down in earnest now.

I had a feeling the rehearsals were over.

Eighty

At 5:50pm, Jeffrey needed morphine and suctioning, and the marathon began.

6:45pm—morphine and suctioning

6:55pm—ditto

7:05pm—ditto

7:15pm—ditto

7:20pm—ditto

7:25pm—ditto

The relentless regimen of morphine and suctioning forced me on autopilot more than ever. Morphine/suction/morphine/suction. I feared there might not be an end to this nightmarish gerbil wheel, and that if there was, I wouldn't recognize it… or be able to get off if I tried.

7:35pm—more morphine. The morphine was not doing its job. Jeffrey seemed to be in distress even under the influence, and nothing I did eased it.

DEAR GOD, PLEASE TAKE HIM!!!

As soon as Randy returned home from delivering Katie to the Brownie meeting at school, he called Mary to see how much additional morphine Jeffrey could tolerate. She gave him the adjusted schedule and told him what we should watch for with the adjusted dosage and when to call her again, reminding us she was available if we needed her. I was grateful to know she could come, but I still wanted to keep this an intimate, family-only affair if possible. I prayed continuously for strength to deal with and accept what appeared to be the final lap in Jeffrey's earthly journey.

Just a little longer, surely, and he would be free.

Randy left to pick Katie up from Brownies and rushed straight home. The thought that we were all together provided a sense of security for whatever the evening might bring. It looked promising as an evening of action in some capacity.

7:45pm—morphine

8:00pm—ditto

8:10pm—increased morphine

8:25pm—ditto

8:40pm—ditto

9:00pm—more morphine. By this dose, I was freakishly calm. It had been thirteen hours since I had been out of the chair. Jeffrey's body felt cooler to the touch, and Randy turned the ceiling fan off.

9:25pm—more morphine

9:45pm—more morphine. Matthew, who had spent the evening jabbering nervously, lapsed into the safety of exhaustive sleep on the couch. Randy was upstairs on the phone, updating Nell, and I trusted Katie had crashed in someone's bed at some point. Jeffrey was saturated with morphine, and still he fought the urge to close his eyes… possibly forever. I needed to stretch my body, but I was afraid I would collapse on my wobbly legs. I was also afraid to move Jeffrey even if I thought I *could* move for fear of adding to his apparent distress, and I was certainly afraid to leave him, even for a period of seconds.

I was afraid to blink.

Eighty-one

The sense of urgency continued.

10:15pm—more morphine

10:40pm—Jeffrey's breathing began slowing down, down, down… almost to a stop. My heart raced, as if trying to compensate, or perhaps recharge him. Or perhaps simply because I felt certain that this time, there would be no turning back.

10:42pm—it struck me that while Jeffrey was ready for the final stretch of his transition to eternal safety, he might be holding out because of concern for us. I'd asked God to take him a few times, but I'd never thought to tell Jeffrey himself, to give him permission, other than my feeble mumbling a few weeks before. I'd read that sometimes, that's what it takes.

Cashing in once again on the strength and courage for which I'd prayed relentlessly over the past few months, I looked into Jeffrey's weary eyes and told him to go on, that we would be fine, that we loved him and were so proud he was part of our family, and that we would never forget to appreciate all he had brought and would leave behind for us and so many others.

10:43pm—Jeffrey took two final breaths, as if to say, "Thank you," and officially earned the angel wings that had been waiting for him for 5-1/2 months. He was taken to heaven just as we had prayed, with all of us at home… and peacefully.

Our assignment as Jeffrey's earth family had ended.

Eighty-two

In a combined state of shock, numbness, and (mostly) relief, I could do no more than simply stare at this beautiful baby angel who had endured so much and yet had maintained grace, dignity, and the ability to smile... something we should all strive to possess. In what seemed simultaneously like forever and mere instants, it ended... Jeffrey's distress, our worries for him, our hopes and dreams that we would somehow outwit the killer instincts of SMA.

Direct battle against such a destructive disease had ceased, but we did not have to admit defeat. I refused to let SMA claim victory for Jeffrey's earthly departure and rationalized my feelings with the knowledge that he was safe, happy, healthy, and free forever, and that nothing could harm him again. He had escaped the death clutches of SMA and was in the perfect place. Our love and admiration for him and for God would only intensify, and while we wouldn't be holding him any more, at least for a while, SMA couldn't touch him, either. No, we would not admit defeat.

The tears flowed profusely, of course, but they were mostly tears for Jeffrey's freedom and the realization that we didn't have to worry about him or question our competency anymore. I couldn't believe how calm I felt and how overpowering the feeling of relief was—more so than any emotion I had ever felt, including the sheer ecstasy of giving birth. I would never wish such an experience on anyone, but the feeling of peace and the opportunity to witness the power of faith and prayer was a different matter.

I called Randy, who came downstairs immediately, and told him it was over. His tears also flowed with sadness that Jeffrey was gone but relief that he was now safe. He solemnly turned off the oxygenator for the first time in almost a month; the resulting quiet, unfamiliar to us the previous few months, was deafening. As Randy went back upstairs to phone Nell again and relay the news, I sat with Jeffrey, unable to think in any capacity, in complete disbelief that our assignment was over… or that it had happened in the first place.

When Randy returned downstairs moments later, he once again performed impressively on the phone, calling Paul first, then my folks. Mary was next, and he asked that she allow us forty-five minutes to talk to Matthew and Katie, who were both still fully unconscious in the safety of sleep.

I managed somehow to rise from the Jeffrey chair, place our official angel gently on his pillow in our chair, and head to the bathroom. I had been a fixture in the Jeffrey chair for fourteen hours straight, and I staggered like a zombie.

Once upright, I was grateful my legs remembered how to function and where to go without any conscious guidance on my part, as reality had begun dribbling in. Relieved as I was with Jeffrey's safety from harm, my heart and soul were in shambles.

We were still here.

Eighty-three

I returned to the living room for Jeffrey so I could give him his first real bath and shampoo in weeks before waking Matthew and Katie. He was so perfectly formed, so delicate, so thin. Katie had asked much earlier to help with his final bath, but I decided against letting her see him naked. SMA had erased all evidence of chubby, cuddly baby fat, leaving little more than skin and bones.

Ironically, that probably helped me as I bathed him. There had been such a dramatic change in his appearance over the past few days, it was almost as if we were caring for someone else's baby.

Actually, we were.

Without fear of Jeffrey's going into respiratory distress, I didn't have to rush through the bath, which, surprisingly, I found quite easy. I couldn't have hurried, anyway, as I was functioning in a dream-like slow motion on top of feeling responsible for the final prepping of an angel.

And I knew that once I finished, the next move was to hand him over to the funeral home. No matter that it was just his body. It was our baby's body.

I cut off some of Jeffrey's Elvis hair and placed it inside a baggie, then rubbed sweet baby lotion all over him before putting on a new diaper and the gown from Jaymie. It swallowed him, but he did look like 'the angel that he was.' Simply stunning.

When I finished, satisfied, I placed Jeffrey gently in the cradle in the living room. Randy roused Matthew from the couch and guided his sleepy self upstairs so we could awaken Katie. By then, Mom and Dad had already arrived, ready to tackle whatever chores needed to be done in their own 'relief/grief' phase. They wisely decided to start with the no-brainer of cleaning the kitchen, which would keep them occupied for a while.

I briefly considered how difficult it must have been for my folks and Nell to deal with this double whammy. They endured the agony of losing a grandbaby while watching their own children endure the agony of losing a child. My folks had had the advantage of being around Jeffrey, though, while Nell had had to deal with it from halfway across the country. It was a situation definitely not for wimps, as Mom had said.

I realized I was uttering prayers of thanks for everything— for Jeffrey's release, for Matthew and Katie, for Randy, for our families, for Mary, for our friends and countless unidentifiable others who had provided us with so much support and prayer strength throughout this whole journey.

And there were many thankful prayers to God for His role. He had obviously listened to our pleas and responded, even in those times when we wondered if there were answers, and certainly in times when the answers were not what we wanted to hear. He had not failed in His promise to stay with us, and we knew He would accompany us on the next leg of the journey as well. And the next.

All we had to do was ask.

Eighty-four

Upstairs, we shared the news with Matthew and Katie. Their sadness, magnified by fatigue, was mixed with a mature sense of relief for Jeffrey. We eventually went back downstairs and began the next phase of the Jeffrey journey. Or now, rather, the Jeffrey-less journey in the physical sense. Matthew and Katie jabbered like magpies, unusual not for Katie, but for Matthew. Mary arrived to take care of business, including taking final information and dumping out the remaining morphine. She commented that I looked different standing up, that she had never seen me out of the chair in her visits.

I was in awe of the emotions that consumed me and my ability to function in a capacity that might have almost passed as normal to the untrained eye. While I could have sat and bawled without any provocation, I found myself both calm and giddy, searching anywhere for signs of humor and memories of normalcy. The overwhelming numbness, shock, disbelief, and sense of loss ingrained originally at the time of diagnosis were intense, but even greater was the assurance that Jeffrey was free and safe.

Gary, from the funeral home, whom Randy had also called at some point during the night, unbeknownst to me, was to arrive for Jeffrey or, as Mary repeatedly stated, Jeffrey's *body*. Mary suggested we (except for Randy) stay in the kitchen when Gary arrived, and I didn't argue. When he appeared at the door, I handed a blanket to Randy for Jeffrey because the night was chilly, but Gary had brought one. I knew it must have been tough for him, figuring that he had probably planned to have his own children one day. I wondered if this had altered his thinking.

Gary told Randy the service had already been scheduled for

3:30 Thursday afternoon in order to accommodate the teachers at Mountain View School, who had been so unconditionally supportive from the beginning. The service, as requested by us, would be short and sweet. It didn't take Gary long to prepare Jeffrey's body for the ride to the funeral home, and I actually survived it... but only because I distracted most of myself with conversation in the kitchen. Randy, with his usual remarkable poise, bid Gary—and Jeffrey—good-bye.

We had seen Jeffrey in the earthly sense for the last time. He was now an angel.

Officially.

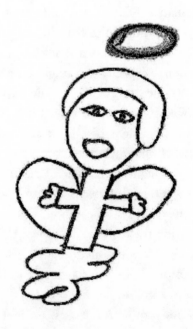

Eighty-five

My folks and Mary eventually headed home, leaving our physically-downsized family to deal with ourselves. Our first task utilizing the surge of adrenaline was to clean the suction machines (the 'death machines,' as Katie had dubbed them), destined for removal as soon as possible. As an excuse to avoid the moments of silence before exhaustion-induced collapse set in, we continued readying the equipment for pickup and cleaning and straightening up for the visitors we anticipated over the next few days.

The need for all of us to talk and hug and remember and assure ourselves that we had done all we could for Jeffrey was undeniable, and sleep would wait, anyway. The longer we talked about the blessings from Jeffrey's unexplained arrival and premature departure, however, the more my numbness dissipated, and the louder the searing hole in my heart screamed. The tears accompanying the enormous lump in my throat refused to be unleashed, but I knew they would spill out soon. Or at least I hoped they would.

Without the ongoing whir, buzz, and sucking sounds of the medical equipment, the silence was painful and served as a hearty reminder of what had just transpired, as hard as it was to believe.

Matthew and Katie finally reached enough emotional and physical fatigue to go back to sleep, but before they crawled into their beds, we looked out at the sky a final time, wondering where Jeffrey was and what he was doing. The stars, always magnificently brilliant in the clear mountain skies, were truly brighter than we'd ever noticed them before, and we spied a wondrous twinkling from one.

We decided it was God's Welcoming Center for Angels, and that Jeffrey must have arrived, safe and sound. And happy. Amen.

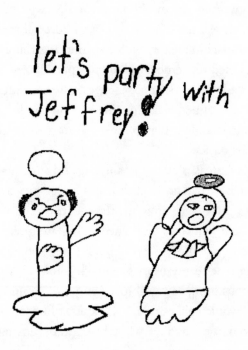

Eighty-six

Most of November 5 was devoted to sharing the announcement with those who had followed our journey closely and to running obligatory errands before Jeffrey's service the following afternoon. Our functioning was purely automatic, as we welcomed friends throughout the day and the arrival of Paul, Jaymie, Jonathan, and Bethany that evening.

Into the early hours of November 6, the day of Jeffrey's send-off, my dozing didn't last long. I lay in bed wondering how I could possibly contribute to the service for Jeffrey. There would be no viewing or open casket, no videos or balloons, and no one in the family would get up and speak of how wonderful Jeffrey's life was here on earth. It *was*… but we wouldn't be able to talk.

Even though the Bible speaks of rejoicing death, I found it incredible that some folks were actually able to do it. I felt immense relief that Jeffrey was free, but how in the world did anyone ever feel like rejoicing a child's death? How did anyone ever feel like rejoicing anything again? I wanted desperately to believe that time was a healer like everyone claimed. We would see.

At 5am, I was drawn out of bed and to the computer downstairs, as the words, *Dear Heavenly Father*, drifted into my consciousness. I began typing words that flowed effortlessly with the tears from my heart, and a letter to God was penned…

Dear Heavenly Father,
In the springtime, when life always seems so hopeful with abundant rejuvenation, You graciously gave our family a priceless gift. We named him Jeffrey and loved him more than we thought possible. We knew he was special from the beginning, and yet in time You

showed us that he was even more special than we imagined. Our love for him intensified and began spilling over into increased love and appreciation for others and for You.

In the fall, when Your brilliant colors and crystal skies defy description, we gave Your gift back to you; not because we wanted to part with him, but because we loved him that much and because You seemed satisfied we had taken good care of him during his brief stay on earth. You chose to accept him on a day when he was surrounded by so many of his loved ones, and You chose the peace and beauty of the night to welcome him back home. It was no coincidence, we know, that the stars were even more magnificent than ever that night…

Because of Your generosity in allowing us to care for Jeffrey, we learned not only about him and his special needs, but more about You, ourselves, and others. We have been reminded just how unique each and every one of us is and how blessed we all are to be part of Your plan. We also more fully appreciate Your own sacrifice to us so long ago.

And so we rejoice with You and thank You for sharing Jeffrey with us and for being with us every step of this incredible journey. We may not be able to hold Jeffrey in our arms now, but we shall hold him in our hearts forever and ever. You have enriched not only the lives of our family beyond comprehension, but also those of countless others who have been touched in some way by Your new angel. We are all richer because of it…

Where these words came from, I had no idea. Because of our Jeffrey journey, however, I had become wholly aware that with God's intervention and my faith in His love, both unwavering, I would never again question the ability of my entire self to rise to the occasion.

Any occasion.

♥

Now... there is a tiny angel
Breathing deep of heaven's air
Whose wings soar out behind him
as he dips and swirls with flare.

There is a tiny angel
Who twinkles in a star
Whose breath is in a mountain breeze
that blows in from afar.

There is a tiny angel
Who flutters softly by
On butterfly wings you'll find him
or in clouds across the sky.

There is a tiny angel
Who has now become a part
Of the love you feel inside you
as you keep him in your heart.

excerpt from 'A Tiny Angel'
by Ravelle Whitener
November, 1997

Epilogue...

Epilogue

As anticipated, the service for Jeffrey was an opportunity to hit rock bottom in this surreal, whirlwind journey, and we did it with ease. My mental picture of Jeffrey's lying in a box didn't register anywhere close to the unbearable anguish at seeing the tiny white casket itself, closed and surrounded by flowers, teddy bears, and pictures of our beaming angel. On top of the excruciating visual torture, we managed to endure a seemingly endless acknowledgment that our baby was really gone and really inside that tiny white box (Randy informed me later that the service, as promised, had lasted twelve minutes). At least we hadn't volunteered to speak as many bereaved parents do, as it would have been impossible. The weather for the service—chilly, gray, and drizzly—was fitting.

Faithful friends joined our family for Jeffrey's official farewell, and the opportunity following the service to thank and hug them for all they had done was the first positive step on the new path of our journey. That part was actually easy.

The graveside mini-service and prayer on top of our little mountain, made possible by the 'Jeffrey' road, was attended by family and close friends. It was much easier to bear than the formal service, thanks to the pensive walk up the mountain, a beautiful sunset replacing the gloomy funeral weather, and a stunning view from Jeffrey's spot… and the fact that one simply cannot sink much further after a child's funeral. Particularly when the child is your own.

Afterwards, as the big folks gathered in the kitchen to nibble on the variety of edibles provided by earth angels, Katie quietly gathered all the pictures of Jeffrey that had been displayed at the service *and* all the flowers and took them upstairs to her small room, rendering it a shrine of sorts to Jeffrey. And then she provided a bit of diversion, before anyone had ~~escaped~~ left, with a show-n-tell of a bloody paper towel bearing her freshly-yanked tooth. Welcome back to the real world!

Life gradually continued falling into place even as the remnants of the protective shell of numbness and shock began disintegrating for good. To say it was smooth sailing would stretch the truth considerably; however, there was plenty of positive motion, thanks to the primary incentive of steering Matthew and Katie forward, and the never-ending reminder to ourselves that Jeffrey was free, safe, and happy.

A brief trip to Pigeon Forge, Tennessee, land of neon, arcades, go-carts, and shopping (but not colleges, as Matthew hoped upon our arrival!), followed a stop at Bethany's wildly-stimulating bowling birthday party two days after Jeffrey's funeral. It was a terrific healing opportunity for all of us, especially Matthew and Katie, and it provided a hint that we could—*would*—find joy again without Jeffrey in our physical midst.

Fast forward a few years… Randy returned to high school teaching and coaching, still entertaining fans and outwitting opposing coaches with creative offensive game plans and making a difference for many students. Matthew returned to his alma mater to work on his master's in education while helping coach his former football teammates. He is on the verge of graduating, as is Katie, a photography major snagging her diploma a year ahead of schedule. All are pretty wonderful!

~

Jeffrey's body left us behind, but his spirit most certainly didn't. The first no-doubt-about-it Jeffrey sign occurred less than two months after his death. With Nellie in tow, we all walked up the mountain in the middle of a beautiful, heavy snow. The skies had been gloomy and gray all day with no signs of the snow's letting up, but as we were determined to go up to Jeffrey's site, we bundled up and did. At the precise moment we set our frozen feet on the mountain top, the gray clouds opened up to reveal a gorgeous clear blue sky. We looked at each other in awe and said a prayer at Jeffrey's site before heading back. As soon as we set foot off the top of the mountain (out of site of Jeffrey's spot), the blue disappeared behind the gray... and stayed that way for the remainder of the day.

Other signs, which still pop up to our delight, have included both 'timely' appearances of wild critters and gorgeous birds in the yard (and closer!) and rainbows at unexpected times, impromptu bursts of sunshine on gloomy days when I need a boost of sorts, blooming of previously uncooperative plants around Jeffrey's birthday or angel day... and the the list goes on. These moments still ease the emptiness when Jeffrey is particularly missed and are always welcomed reminders that he is fine. And, by the grace of God, so are we. After the death of my father (who has left his own signs!), it's easy to imagine their plotting 'reminders' together!

Thanks to Jeffrey (and Dad!), 'coincidences' are now referred to as Angel Intervention. I wish I had time to keep track of the evidence, but the angel brigade doesn't take many breaks!

From the beginning of the grief process, which started at the diagnosis, there was plenty of backsliding to what felt like the proverbial square one, but that is part of grief and grieving, a bizarre and immensely torturous process at best. It takes time and patience—a bundle of both—to muddle through the quicksand of despair, and while I know there are folks who don't believe prayer is beneficial, I don't know how they function without it.

Although it has been over twelve years since our active Jeffrey assignment, we realized just how close to the surface the memories remain when my father's health began declining during the early spring of 2006 until his death a few short months later. Although we weren't dealing with SMA this time, the similarities between the situations were uncanny in many ways, making some aspects of our Papa assignment more difficult, others slightly easier. The most comforting vision of all continues to be the one of Jeffrey and his beloved Papa making up for lost time by sharing guffaws… a lot.

∼

Despite the end of the first stretch of the Jeffrey journey, the journey itself forges on. The battle against SMA is waged now on behalf of not only the memory of Jeffrey, but also for Matthew and Katie and their children, our nieces and nephews and their children, and for all others in the SMA family.

Researchers focusing solely on SMA continue to advance towards the finish line with incredible speed and optimism (see *SMA Research & Outlook* in the following section, **Facts About SMA**). It is predicted that a viable cure for SMA can be reached within five years. FIVE.

The price tag for the continuation of research is staggering; however, it will never override the passion, tenacity, and courage of families around the world who face head-on the demands of SMA in order to obliterate its status as a genetic nightmare. Indeed, these families seem to thrive on clearing hurdles insurmountable to most. Fundraising activities by families and their supporters to increase awareness of SMA and their own angels and to help fund research and families' needs are creative, industrious, heartwarming, insanely successful, and more than a little therapeutic.

~

In addition to raising funds for research, SMA families have assumed increasing responsibility in devising individual programs for their children in such areas as diet and noninvasive treatment when warranted. Dr. John R. Bach, whose name was only beginning to emerge during our Jeffrey days, is sought out for his interest, expertise, dedication, and established non-invasive protocol in the management of neuromuscular and pulmonary disease. He is joined by a growing number of competent and caring comrades in the field, several of whom are conducting extremely encouraging trials.

Doctors in general still lack sufficient knowledge of the disease, and, in some frustrating cases, seem reluctant to learn; however, a shift in knowledge and attitude among the medical pros is inevitable, given the persistent efforts of SMA families and the increasing number of physicians drawn into the world of SMA for one reason or another.

~

The support among families, each battling their own ever-present trials and tribulations, is indescribable. Incomprehensible, actually. The camaraderie among the members of the SMA family, with their common goal of providing the best for their children's well-being, is both understandable and unique in that the bulk of the hugs, tears, advice, and news bulletins, encouraging and otherwise, is accomplished solely through the avenues of technology. Indeed, access to the wonders of the Internet for information and contact with fellow warriors should be made readily available to anyone dealing with such devastation.

Supplementing organizational chapters, there is a growing

trend towards 'reunion' meetings of families, providing bonding opportunities for parents and children alike that transcend even the most Kodak® of moments.

Opportunities for families to spread the word to the outside world have also increased by leaps and bounds with a few creative endeavors in the mix. Some years ago, SMA parents representing two families spent a frigid thirty-six hours atop the JVC billboard in Times Square to raise funds and awareness. During that stint, a few SMA families were able to contact Rosie O'Donnell, who graciously posted the Families of SMA number on the screen and on the backs of all the seats in the audience of the show she hosted at the time. In early 2004, an SMA parent and two researchers perched atop the Hershey's Chocolate Building in Times Square, spreading SMA awareness to passersby and chocolate to donors.

It's not just families in overdrive when it comes to getting the word out. One of the most memorable 'layman' stories involves Thomas Becker, a decorated veteran, recreational bowler, and former bowling alley manager. In 1998, after visiting a local baby with SMA whose story he'd seen on TV, he decided to draw attention to SMA via himself as a marathon bowler, determined to break the most strenuous bowling record in the *Guinness Book of World Records*. After 25 hours of continuous bowling, Thomas had a new world record... and dehydration, exhaustion, and agonizing raw blisters on his hands and feet, requiring a trip to the hospital. Six weeks later, baby Allie earned her official wings, prompting Becker to commit to an even more industrious feat—bowling in all 50 states in 100 days. He became the world's only marathon bowler, enduring 'infinity' blisters and profuse gratitude in order to increase awareness and raise funds on behalf of SMA.

Today there are countless individuals working on behalf of those with SMA. *Countless* meaning it's impossible to keep up with them all!

Those with SMA are making quite a bit of noise themselves. In the now defunct magazine, *Rosie* (August, 2001), the Editor's Letter page highlighted a ten-year old girl with SMA who designs beautiful greeting cards as a fundraiser for SMA research. In *YM* (*Your Magazine*, October, 2001), one of my two distant cousins with SMA was featured in a Make-A-Wish makeover by *YM*.

The late Nicki Ard, Ms. Wheelchair America 2001, had SMA and was always willing and eager to promote awareness and help the cause however she could. Kristen Connors, Ms. Wheelchair America 2006, has SMA, as does Melissa Milinovich, the third runner-up and Ms. Wheelchair Ohio 2005. Lindsey Muszkiewicz was chosen by Milkbone to appear on boxes as a spokesperson for Canine Assistants. Morgan Fritz replaced the late Mattie Stepanek as the 2005 MDA National Goodwill Ambassador and was followed by Luke Christie, the two-time MDA National Goodwill Ambassador. Both have SMA.

In July, 2009, Morgan Kelly, 11, placed second in the Pre-teen America Nationals, Senior Division. She was the youngest to place in that division, earning second in Senior Speech and Best Overall Interview, Top 20, and Pre-teen America Spirit of Pre-teen Senior. Not bad for a rising 6th-grader. I was still playing with dolls at that age.

The heartwarming documentary, *39 Pounds of Love*, follows 34-year old Ami Ankilewitz, a 3D animator with the function of a single finger, as he crossed the United States in search of the doctor who had issued a prognosis of 'death by age six' to Ami's mother. The poignant story of his adventure won the Israeli Oscar; in Hollywood, it was presented with a Media Access Award and was screened by the Academy of Motion Pictures Arts and Sciences as part of their 'outstanding documentaries' series. Ami's generosity was instrumental in forming Ami's Angels Foundation, the goal of which was to enhance the lives of disabled youth through technology. Sadly for the rest of us, Ami passed away in September, 2009. He was 41.

Keep your eyes on two particularly bright young adults in the SMA family, Margaret (MJ) Purk and Victor Alvarez. Both began their college careers with impressive credentials, including a Volvo for Life award for MJ and a Bill Gates scholarship for Victor. Thankfully, they didn't listen to their doctors' gloomy predictions, either, and continue providing encouragement and inspiration to SMA families with babies and children as well as forcing their able-bodied college peers to rise up to their standards. Wish their peers luck.

∼

Witnessing the expansion of SMA recognition in myriad ways raises high hopes that our collective efforts to heighten awareness are paying off. States across the country have joined forces in proclaiming August 'SMA Awareness Month.' Students in college and high school (including a niece, one of my former students, and Katie) have selected SMA as the topic of their research projects, utilizing vital input from families themselves. Various annual conferences provide invaluable opportunities for families, physicians, and researchers to congregate and share accomplishments, questions, advice, goals, and dreams.

Media has helped ignite the cause. In early 2001, ABC News' *UpClose* spotlighted SMA and the dire need for additional funding. Celebrities, their clout considered the golden key to essential funding for worthy causes, are speaking up on behalf of SMA families. Howie Long, well-known for his athletic endeavors and quick wit, served for several years as the spokesperson for Andrew's Buddies/Fight SMA. Gary Sinise and Jeff Perry, both respected actors and directors, created a Public Service Announcement for

Discovery Channel Radio, CNN, and other radio stations to raise awareness of SMA and Families of SMA. In addition, actors David Duchovny and Tea Leoni served as honorary chairpersons of the Cure SMA Walk-n-Roll Across America.

MDA Celebrity Ambassadors, designated to help draw attention to muscular dystrophy in general, include television's Alison Sweeney (*Days of Our Lives*, *The Biggest Loser*) and Brandon Barash (*General Hospital*), along with singers Billy Gilman and Ace Young, an American Idol semifinalist. Nancy O'Dell (formerly of *Access Hollywood*) is the MDA's National ALS Ambassador, working passionately in memory of her mother.

Additional celebrities bolstering the cause with actual ties to SMA include Traci Bingham (whose niece had SMA), Teddy Geiger (with a family connection), and Don Davis of the New England Patriots (whose cousin had SMA). The cane used by Hugh Laurie during the first season of *House, M.D.* was auctioned off to raise funds for SMA on behalf of the son of Garrett Lerner, executive producer/writer. In one episode of *House*, 'spinal muscular atrophy' was mentioned in passing by a young patient, while in another, the main character had SMA.

In 2005 and again in 2008, *Extreme Makeover: Home Edition* selected an SMA family for its incredible dreams-do-come-true makeovers.

Music groups have also been rocking on behalf of various SMA organizations. O.A.R., a 'reggae and roots-rock jam band,' hails from Ohio, home to significant SMA research efforts. They have generously assisted charitable organizations by matching donations received on their tours, selecting SMA (Miracle for Madison and Friends) as an early recipient of their goodwill. Members of the band, Widespread Panic, have donated time and money doing benefits on behalf of Andrew's Buddies. The Dixie Chicks' Martie Maguire became involved with an SMA family and requested that gifts honoring the arrival of her twins in 2004 be in the form of donations to Families of SMA.

And we are now racing to a cure… literally. Jimmie Johnson, race car driver, selected Families of SMA as one of the two final charities to grace a spot on his Helmet of Hope for the Sprint Cup series on October 11, 2009. The fact that he crossed the finish line first (again!) is heartily cheered by his fans, old and new.

~

Foundations set up by families abound in all corners of the world. Some focus on awareness and research funding. Others set their sights towards helping families whose needs for critical equipment and miscellaneous supplies often fall through relentlessly stubborn and maddeningly senseless insurance cracks.

Local affiliates of Families of SMA and Fight SMA are peppered across the country, uniting families in fundraising and awareness efforts while providing valuable support for all. Online networking, such as Facebook, Twitter, and SMASpace, continue opening doors far beyond our imagination. Well, mine, anyway. It was largely the miracle of cyberspace elves that helped propel The Jennifer Trust for SMA to top spot in the 2009 National Lottery Award in Best Health category, and then there's the Gwendolyn Strong Foundation (more about them coming up!).

Liaisons between volunteer groups associated with various SMA-focused organizations and representatives in Washington have been stirring up enthusiasm and interest in strategic places. Dr. Duane Alexander, Director of the National Institute of Child Health & Development, committed to actively supporting SMA as part of the newborn screening initiative. In addition, NIH identified SMA as the disease closest to 600 others, meaning that a cure for SMA will bring a cure within reach for close to 600 other diseases, such as ALS, Parkinson's, Alzheimer's, Duchenne muscular dystrophy, and Tay-Sachs.

In a strategic move forward is the SMA Treatment Acceleration Act of 2009 (H.R. 2149/S. 1158), introduced in the U.S. House of Representatives by Congressmen Patrick Kennedy (D-RI) and Eric Cantor (R-VA) and in the U.S. Senate by Senators Debbie Stabenow (D-MI) and Johnny Isakson (R-GA). In a quest to encourage further support in Washington, Bill and Victoria Strong, parents to Gwendolyn and founders of the Gwendolyn Strong Foundation, initiated the online Petition to Cure SMA, with an original goal of 1000 signatures, which are steadily closing in on the revised 100,000 mark. Thanks to cyberspace and a few skills(!), they then initiated the unbelievably simple Tweet for a Cure (gwendolynstrongfoundation.org/twitter) to help folks urge their reps to support the SMA Treatment Acceleration Act.

The aptly-named Strong family was hardly finished. Their mission to defeat SMA's wrath through raising awareness and funding for research continued with Sponsor-A-Mile, Shop-ToEndSMA, and Unite for a Cure, which alone raised over $146,000 for research through the collective efforts of numerous motivated families.

And the Strongs continued. Perhaps the most telling example of tenacity, dedication, and absolute passion in the SMA family, coupled with the awesomeness of the Internet, comes from the Chase Community Giving Campaign on Facebook in January, 2010. Over 500,000 charitable organizations entered the campaign with dreams of the top $1 million prize. Only 100 would make it to the finals, earning $25,000 each for their respective charities for the accomplishment. The Gwendolyn Strong Foundation reached the finals; Bill and Victoria couldn't get the check for $25,000 to Dr. Keirstead and his research fast enough. And it wasn't over.

Competing against the big boys in the world of worthy causes, the GSF united not only those in the immediate SMA family but thousands (over 52,000, in fact) outside it. Countless folks spent hours upon hours online in various capacities for a week, in awe of the support from all over—celebrities and supporters of other causes included. And in the end, the Gwendolyn Strong Foundation found itself in the hard-fought 6th place, garnering an additional $100,000 for Dr. Keirstead's impressive, encouraging work and respect for the 'mom & pop' foundation from around the world. Equally important, it raised awareness in ways we may never comprehend.

SMA folks mean business.

All activities devoted to the elimination and/or management of SMA and to heightening awareness are significant and crucial. When the announcement is made of a cure or treatment protocol, its success will likely hinge upon pre-symptomatic intervention.

With only rare exception, however, we are typically unaware of the destructive potential we harbor; unless our own children are diagnosed, we will remain (momentarily) blissfully, and dangerously, ignorant. Until mandatory prenatal screening includes an SMA component, only those who know from devastating experience that they carry the defective gene will know to be vigilant during pregnancy and prepared at birth.

Carrier testing is available now, yet how many without some sort of prior introduction to SMA would know to inquire about it? Possibly none.

The insistence on continued research, education, awareness, and funding will therefore linger way beyond the pronouncement of a 'cure.' We will battle SMA as long and as diligently as necessary... grateful for every accomplishment along the way, but not content until SMA is history.

~

Thank you for any interest you may have acquired in helping us defuse this genetic time bomb. With your assistance, whether it be from sharing this journey with others, making monetary donations to an SMA group (see the first section in **Guide to Helpful Resources**), supporting a local fundraiser, urging your senators and representatives to support the SMA Treatment Acceleration Act, and/or including a specific or entire SMA family in your prayers, you are making a difference in the quest of many.

You won't regret it.

Facts About SMA
Research & Outlook
Guide to Helpful Resources

What is Spinal Muscular Atrophy?

Courtesy of
Families of SMA, SMA Coalition, and SMA Support

Spinal muscular atrophy (SMA) is a genetic disease caused by deletions and/or mutations in the survival motor neuron gene 1 (SMN1). This SMN1 gene is responsible for the production of a protein essential to the proper functioning of the motor neurons, which are nerve cells in the spinal cord that send signals to muscles throughout the body. People with SMA are missing both copies of SMN1, while carriers are missing only one.

Without the critical SMN protein, the nerve cells atrophy (wither) and eventually die, resulting in weakness of the muscles used for crawling, sitting, walking, head and neck control, sucking, and swallowing. Respiratory muscles are also affected.

There are several types of SMA; typically, the earlier the diagnosis, the more severe the SMA. Type 1, usually diagnosed within the first two months, is the most severe; typical infant milestones are never reached. Intelligence is not affected in any type; in fact, those with SMA are often noted to be unusually bright and sociable.

A baby must inherit the SMA gene from both carrier parents in order to have SMA. If the defective gene is passed from only one parent, the baby will be a carrier but will not have SMA. If neither parent passes on the defective gene, the baby will not have SMA or be a carrier.

A more detailed explanation of SMA and descriptions of the various types may be located on several SMA web sites, including Families of SMA, SMA Coalition, SMA Support, and Spinal Muscular Atrophy Foundation (see Guide to Helpful Resources page).

Quick Facts About SMA

Courtesy of
Families of SMA, Fight SMA,
Miracle for Madison and Friends, SMA Coalition,
and Spinal Muscular Atrophy Foundation

**SMA is the number one genetic killer of children
under the age of two.**

**As many as one in 35-40 people are carriers
of the SMA gene**
(approximately 7 million people).

As many as one in 6,000 babies born annually worldwide
are afflicted with some form of SMA. This is similar to
the incidence of Tay Sachs (in the Jewish population) and
Duchenne muscular dystrophy.

At least 50% of children diagnosed with SMA before the age of
2 will likely die before their second birthday.

The chance that both parents are carriers is as great as
1 in 1,600.

For EACH pregnancy with two carrier parents, there is a:
50% chance that the baby will be a carrier,
25% chance that the baby will have SMA,
25% chance that the baby will be SMA-free.

It is believed that over 25,000 Americans have some form of SMA. The prevalence of SMA is comparable to that of amyotrophic lateral sclerosis (ALS, or Lou Gehrig's Disease) and cystic fibrosis.

There are no race, gender, or age boundaries with SMA.

SMA Research & Outlook

Courtesy of
Families of SMA, SMA Coalition, and SMA Foundation

Dramatic breakthroughs in the past fifteen years, such as the discovery of the SMN1 gene and its production of the protein critical to the health of motor neurons, have transformed SMA from an obscure disease to one on the threshold of treatment.

One particularly exciting discovery is that of a partially- functioning backup copy of SMN1 called SMN2, which people with SMA possess even in the absence of SMN1. Research is focused on drugs and genetic therapies that appear likely to enhance the capabilities of SMN2; the greater the amount of functional SMN protein produced by SMN2, the more motor neurons can be supported and kept healthy. Scientists have already identified drugs that appear promising and are now in the process of testing these leads in trials.

Scientists now believe SMA may have a greater probability of realizing treatment or cure than any other major genetic disease. Because it offers a high probability of developing treatment or cure, is relatively common *(particularly interesting since it is still considered rare by many in the medical profession)*, is a devastating children's disease, and has no current treatment, it has been selected by NIH as a model for a new approach to funding translational research. It doesn't hurt that the cure for SMA will benefit approximately 600 other diseases, including ALS, Alzheimer's, Parkinson's, Duchenne muscular dystrophy, and Tay Sachs.

Translational research develops ('translates') findings made by scientists in the lab into drugs and treatments that doctors

223

can eventually use to treat patients and, hopefully, save lives. The next step in the program, which is currently proceeding well, is advancing compounds from the SMA translation pilot into clinical trials where they can actually be used by patients. So far, the trials have produced exciting results and hope that the end really is in sight!

Dr. Hans Keirstead's research using stem cells has also produced mind-boggling results and is moving briskly toward human testing.

Development of these treatments within the next few years would likely require $20–30 million of annual research funding, significantly more than the current allotment of funds earmarked for SMA.

The race continues… as do the dreams, determination, and passion of those in the SMA family.

~

To see if your senators/representatives have signed the SMA Treatment Acceleration Act and/or to learn how to contact them, go to www.fightsma.org and click on *Winning on the Hill.*

To encourage your senators/representatives to sign the SMA Treatment Acceleration Act, go to www.thepetitionsite.com/182/petition-to-cure-SMA

Tweet for a Cure— gwendolynstrongfoundation.org/twitter

Guide to Helpful Resources

SMA

Act for SMA—www.actsma.co.uk

Andrew's Buddies/Fight SMA—www.fightsma.com/804-515-0080

Angel Baby Foundation—www.angelbabyfoundation.org

Angel Wings Awareness Quilt—www.kaydence.org/quilt
  (Quilt squares made for 'official' SMA angels)

Dr. John R. Bach—www.doctorbach.com
  Affiliated with UMDNJ-NJ Medical School
    (Deals with patients with neuromuscular disease, pulmonary disease, and home mechanical ventilation)

Blankets for SMA (B4SMA)—www.our-sma-angels.com/b4sma
  (Blankets sent to children with SMA)
  Online store*—www.cafepress.com/b4sma
  *(*SMA Calendar may also be purchased here)*

Claire Altman Heine Foundation, Inc.—
  www.clairealtmanheinefoundation.org

Cole's Quilts—www.our-sma-angels.com/colesquilts
  (Quilts made for SMA babies and children)

Dreams for Jeffrey (CD)—JoAnn Derden—thejeffreyjourney.com
  (JoAnn is Helen's mother/Jeffrey's grandmother; she will soon be releasing more of her original compositions)

Eminnea, Inc.—www.eminnea.org

Fairy Tale (CD)—Alexa Dectis—www.alexadectis.com
  (Alexa has SMA; a portion of the proceeds benefit SMA research)

F.A.M.E. Hispana—espanol.groups.yahoo.com/group/FAME_Hispana/

Families of SMA (FSMA)—www.fsma.org or www.curesma.org
  1-800-886-1762 (US/Canada); 847-367-7620 (all others)

Families of SMA (FSMA)/Type 1 Resources—
  www.fsma.org/FSMACommunity/NewlyDiagnosed/type1/

Fight SMA/Andrew's Buddies—www.fightsma.com/804-515-0080

Fight SMA/Andrew's Buddies Blog—www.fightsma.org/blog

Gray's Gang—www.graysgang.com

(The) Gwendolyn Strong Foundation—
www.gwendolynstrongfoundation.org

Hailey Mae Foundation—www.haileymaefoundation.org

(The) Hope and Light Foundation—www.hopeandlight.org

(The) Jacob Isaac Rappoport Foundation—www.ourshootingstar.com

(The) Jennifer Trust for SMA (JTSMA)—www.jtsma.org.uk

Kennedy's Disease Association—www.kennedysdisease.org

Know SMA—www.knowsma.org

Kyle's Pillow Project—Contact Jana Gundy-mjtgundy@yahoo.com
*(Custom 'positioning' pillows made for children with physical
disabilities; Jana's son, Kyle, has SMA)*

Lucas Was Here—lucaswashere.com

Marshall's Miles—www.marshallsmiles.com

Melissa Milinovich, Ms. Wheelchair Ohio 2005 / 3rd runner-up,
Ms. Wheelchair America 2006—kinsitha@yahoo.com
(Melissa has SMA; she is a child & adult motivator/mentor)

Milverstead Publishing LLC—www.milversteadpublishing.com
*(Chris Finlan, founder, donates a portion of his book's proceeds to the
Gwendolyn Strong Foundation and encourages his authors to donate
to charitable causes)*

Miracle for Madison & Friends—www.miracleformadison.org
(Site of original SMA awareness pin)

Muscular Dystrophy Association (MDA)—www.mdausa.org

Not a Fire Exit—Christopher Finlan—www.notafireexit.com
*(Novel based loosely on SMA family; foreword by Hillary Dunlop
Schmid, SMA mom. Partial proceeds go to the Gwendolyn Strong
Foundation. Available at Amazon.com)*

(The) Olive Branch Fundvwww.theolivebranchfund.org
(Raising funds for pediatric neuromuscular diseases)

Our SMA Angels—www.our-sma-angels.com

Pathways of Promise—www.pathwaysofpromise.org

Paytons Pals—www.paytonspals.com

Petition to Cure SMA—
    www.thepetitionsite.com/182/petition-to-cure-SMA

SMA Angels Charity, Inc.—smaangels.org
    *(Special 'gravity-less' arm slings enabling more independent coloring,
    playing, etc. are made and donated to Type 1 children. See example—
    www.believe-miracles.com)*

SMA Australia—www.smaaustralia.com

SMA Coalition—www.smacoalition.org

SMA Friends—groups.yahoo.com/group/SMAfriends

SMA Medical Supply—www.smasupply.com

SMASpace—smaspace.ning.com

SMA Support—www.smasupport.com / 317-536-6063

(The) SMA Trust (UK)—www.smatrust.org

Song of Dreams (CD)—Jana James—www.cdbaby.com/cd/jamesjana
    (Proceeds benefit SMA Angels Charity, Inc.)

Sophia's Cure—sophiascure.com

Spinal Muscular Atrophy Foundation—www.smafoundation.org

Stop SMA—www.stopsma.org

(The) Suite Life of Lucy and Ethel—
    thesuitelifeoflucyandethel.blogspot.com
    (Blog by Helen and Cindy Schaefer, mom to Kevin, Type 2)

Through Eli's Eyes—througheliseyes.org

Tracy's Story—The Other Side of the Coin—Tracy Armstrong
    *(Milverstead Publishing LLC—released spring, 2010; a portion of
    the proceeds will benefit SMA and MDA causes)*

(The) Wyatt Kyle Sutker Foundation—www.wkswithsma.com

Special Needs—General

Charities/Foundations:

Ace & TJ's Grin Kids—www.grinkids.org

Andrew's Toybox—www.andrewstoybox.org

   (Gina Fimbel's baby, Andrew, had SMA)

CarePages—www.carepages.com

Caring Bridge—www.caringbridge.com

Challenged America—www.challengedamerica.com

(The) Dolan Fund (PA, NJ, DE)—www.dolanfund.org

First Hand Foundation—www.cerner.com/firsthand

Hugs and Hope—www.hugsandhope.org

Jimmie Johnson Foundation—www.jimmiejohnsonfoundation.org

   (Families of SMA was one of two final charities to be chosen for the foundation's 'Helmet of Hope' worn by race car driver, Johnson, during the Sprint Cup Series 10-11-09... which he won!)

Johnathan's Journey*—www.johnathansjourney.org

   Cindi's Photographic Creations—www.cindi-broome.com

   (*Inspired by Johnathan Browning, who had SMA)

Kyle's Pillow Project—Contact Jana Gundy—mjtgundy@yahoo.com

   (Custom 'positioning' pillows made for children with physical disabilities; Jana's son, Kyle, has SMA)

Local Independent Charities—www.lic.org

Make a Child Smile—www.makeachildsmile.org

Make-A-Wish Foundation—www.wish.org

No Boundaries */Muscular Dystrophy Family Foundation*—
   www.noboundariesff.org

   (*<u>Not</u> affiliated w/MDA or Jerry Lewis MDA Labor Day Telethon)

Patient Advocate Foundation—www.patientadvocate.org

Pet Pals of Texas—www.petpalsoftexas.org

   (Vicki Jurney-Taylor, Founder & President, has SMA)

Positive Exposure—www.positiveexposure.org

Ronald McDonald House Charities—rmhc.org
Ryan House—www.ryanhouse.org
    (Holly & Jonathan Cotter's son, Ryan, has SMA)
Songs of Love Foundation—www.songsoflove.org
Special Kids Fund—www.specialkidsfund.org
String of Pearls—www.stringofpearlsonline.com
(The) Sunshine Foundation—www.sunshinefoundation.org
Survival Mode Parent—www.survivalmodeparent.org

Fundraising:
First Giving—www.firstgiving.com
GoodSearch—www.goodsearch.com
iGive.com—www.iGive.com
Milverstead Publishing LLC—www.milversteadpublishing.com
    (Chris Finlan, founder, donates a portion of his book's proceeds to the Gwendolyn Strong Foundation and encourages his authors to donate to charitable causes)

Grief/Loss:
Bereavement Publications, Inc—www.bereavementmag.com
    (Includes info on a variety of online support groups)
Compassion Books—www.compassionbooks.com
(The) Compassionate Friends—www.compassionatefriends.com
Grief: Loss and Recovery (CD)—JoAnn Derden—thejeffreyjourney.com
    (JoAnn is Helen's mother/Jeffrey's grandmother; she will soon be releasing more of her original compositions)
(The) Grieving Garden: Living with the Death of a Child—Suzanne Redfern and Susan K. Gilbert
Grieving Parents—www.grievingparents.com
    (Samantha Stack's daughter, Gabriella, had SMA)
On Grief and Grieving—Elisabeth Kübler-Ross & David Kessler—www.davidkessler.org
String of Pearls—www.stringofpearlsonline.com

Media

Books:

Almost Perfect: Disabled Pets and the People Who Love Them—Ed.—Mary Shafer—www.wordforgebooks.com/almostperfect

(The) Cure: How a Father Raised $100 Million—And Bucked the Medical Establishment—In a Quest to Save His Children—Geeta Anand

(The) Elephant in the Playroom—Denise Brodey

From CP to CPA—Robin Pritts

Lemon the Duck—Laura Backman—www.lemontheduck.com
  (Children's book about a special Pekin duck)

Moonrise: One Family, Genetic Identity, and Muscular Dystrophy—Penny Wolfson

Not a Fire Exit—Christopher Finlan
  (Novel based loosely on SMA family; foreword by Hillary Dunlop Schmid, SMA mom. Partial proceeds go to the Gwendolyn Strong Foundation. Available at Amazon.com)

On a Roll: Reflections from the Wheelchair Dude with the Winning Attitude—Greg Smith (The Strength Coach)
  (Available thru Special Needs Project -www.specialneeds.com)

(The) Other Kid (workbook)—www.theotherkid.com

Shut Up About… Your Perfect Kid!—Gina (Terrasi) Gallagher and Patricia (Terrasi) Konjoian

(The) Squeaky Wheel—Brian Shaughnessy

Teens with the Courage to Give—Jackie Waldman

Thisbe's Promise—Laurian Scott
  (Children's book; Laurian's daughter, Thisbe, had BVVL, a motor neuron disease similar to SMA, as did her son, Noah. Available thru ETS Publishing—www.etspublishinghouse.com)

Weakling Willie—Sabrina Low-DuMond
  (Children's book about muscular dystrophy)

What Adults with Disabilities Wish All Parents Knew, Reflections
from a Different Journey
(Jenn Malatesta & Lisa Bertolini, contributors, have SMA;
available thru disABILITIES Books—www.disabilitiesbooks.com)

Books by Authors with SMA/SMA connections:

Accidental Courage, Boundless Dreams—Amy Jaffe Barzach and San-
dy Tovray Greenberg
(Amy and Peter Barzach's baby, Jonathan, had SMA; Amy also found-
ed Boundless Playgrounds)

Accidents of Nature—Harriet McBryde Johnson

AVOIDING Attendants from HELL—June Price

(The) Best Dancer—Christoph Keller (translated by Alison Gallup)

Death… and the lessons i learned—Louise Smith—
www.TheLessonsofLife.com
(Louise's niece, Rebecca, has SMA)

I Like to Run Too—Stacy Zoern

Jamie: A Literacy Story—Diane Parker
(Diane's student, Jamie, had SMA)

Living with Spinal Muscular Atrophy—Susan Allen and Trina Allen
(Trina's baby/Susan's grandbaby, Kassidy, had SMA)

Marvelous Mercer—Shea Megale—www.marvelousmercer.com

(The) Me in the Mirror—Connie Panzarino

Not a Fire Exit—Christopher Finlan
(Novel based loosely on SMA family; foreword by Hillary Dunlop
Schmid, SMA mom. Partial proceeds go to the Gwendolyn Strong
Foundation. Available at Amazon.com)

(The) Third Opinion—J. Stephen Mikita

Too Late to Die Young—Harriet McBryde Johnson

Tracy's Story—The Other Side of the Coin—Tracy Armstrong
(Milverstead Publishing LLC—released spring, 2010; a portion of
the proceeds will benefit SMA and MDA causes)

<u>Two Fat Mittens</u>—Wanda Wosika and Dona Neubauer
   (Children's book; Wanda's granddaughter, Jessica, has SMA)
<u>VICTORious Life</u>—Elizabeth Jamsa Gearhart
   (About Victor Alvarez, who has SMA—www.victoralvarezweb.com;
   available thru Elizabeth—egearhart@rgv.rr.com)
<u>What Adults with Disabilities Wish All Parents Knew, Reflections from</u>
<u>a Different Journey</u>
   (Jenn Malatesta & Lisa Bertolini, contributors, have SMA; available
   thru disABILITIES Books—www.disabilitiesbooks.com)
<u>What Lies Behind His Eyes</u>—Buddy Bryan
<u>Without Laughter and Music, Shoot Me</u>—Linda Napolitano

Book Sources/Publishing:

Bookshare—www.bookshare.org
DisABILITIES Books—www.disabilitiesbooks.com
Milverstead Publishing LLC—www.milversteadpublishing.com
   (Chris Finlan, founder, donates a portion of his book's proceeds to the
   Gwendolyn Strong Foundation and encourages his authors to donate
   to charitable causes)
Special Needs Project—www.specialneeds.com
Woodbine House (Special-Needs Collection)—woodbinehouse.com

Documentaries/Movies:

Darius Goes West—www.dariusgoeswest.org
Music Within (Based on a true story)—www.musicwithinmovie.com
Shooting Beauty: Everyone Deserves a Shot—
   www.EveryoneDeservesaShot.com
39 Pounds of Love—39poundsoflove.com

Magazines:

Complex Child E-Magazine—www.complexchild.com
Disability World—www.disabilityworld.org

Exceptional Parent Magazine—www.eparent.com

MDA/Quest Magazine—www.mdausa.org/publications/Quest

New Mobility—www.newmobility.com

Ragged Edge Online—www.ragged-edge-mag.com

Wings—Contact Jo D'Archangelis—jodarlis@aol.com
   (Quarterly newsletter focusing on issues of disability, church, and church accessibility; Jo, editor, has SMA)

Music (CD):

Dreams for Jeffrey—JoAnn Derden—thejeffreyjourney.com
   (JoAnn is Helen's mother/Jeffrey's grandmother; she will soon be releasing more of her original compositions)

Fairy Tale—Alexa Dectis—www.alexadectis.com
   (Alexa has SMA; a portion of the proceeds benefit SMA research)

Grief: Loss and Recovery—JoAnn Derden—thejeffreyjourney.com
   (JoAnn is Helen's mother/Jeffrey's grandmother; she will soon be releasing more of her original compositions)

Song of Dreams—Jana James—www.cdbaby.com/cd/jamesjana
   (Proceeds benefit SMA Angels Charity, Inc.)

Visual Arts:

Culture! Disability! Talent!—www.culturedisabilitytalent.org

Icerazer Studios—icerazerstudios.com
   (Nathan Herman, artist, has SMA)

Kerri's Kreations—Web site TBA
   (Kerri Costello, artist, has SMA)

Marina Paskina's Art Gallery—www.mpaskina.com/en
   (Marina, artist, has SMA)

(The) MDA Art Collection—www.mda.org/commprog/art

Positive Exposure—www.positiveexposure.org

Very Special Artists (VSA) Registry—
   www.vsarts.org/prebuilt/artists/registry/artistlisting.cfm

Very Special Arts (VSA)—www.vsarts.org

Whimsical Wildlife & More…—www.KarenWheeler.com

(Karen Wheeler, artist, has SMA)

Willard Wigen—www.willard-wigan.com

Mobility/Travel:

DisabledTravelers.com—www.disabledtravelers.com

Dragon Mobility—www.dragonmobility.com

(Dan Everard, designer, has a daughter, Ruth, with SMA; his son, Sam, had SMA)

Gimp on the Go—www.gimponthego.com

Simplantex—www.simplantex.co.uk

Turbo Owners Club—www.turboownersclub.org.uk

(Ruth Everard, whose dad designed the Everaids Turbo chair, has SMA)

USA TechGuide—www.usatechguide.org

WheelchairGear—www.wheelchairgear.com

Wheelchair Getaways—wheelchairgetaways.com

Wheelchair Junkie.com—www.wheelchairjunkie.com

Wheelchair Recycler, Inc.—www.wheelchair-recycler.com

Wheelchairs and Their Active Users—lenmac.tripod.com

World on Wheelz—www.worldonwheelz.com

Multiple Resource, general:

(The) Boulevard—www.blvd.com

Disability Resource Directory—www.d-r-d.com/disabilityresource.html

DisabilityResources.org—www.disabilityresources.org

Disaboom—www.disaboom.com

GimpGear—www.gimpgear.us

Planet Mobility—www.planetmobility.com

Proyecto Vision—www.proyectovision.net

Online Chat:

MDA—www.mdausa.org/chat/calendar.html
SMA Support—www.smasupport.com/chat_list.htm

Parent/Family:

Brave Kids—www.bravekids.org
ChildrenWeCare4—www.childrenwecare4.com
Families Together for People with Disabilities—
    www.familiestogether.org
Family Support Network of NC—www.fsnnc.org
Family Village—familyvillage.wisc.edu/index.html
(The) Fathers Network—www.fathersnetwork.org
Hopeful Parents—www.hopefulparents.org
KASA (Kids As Self Advocates)—www.fvkasa.org
Moms in Common—www.momsincommon.org
National Inclusion Project—www.inclusionproject.org
NECTAC (National Early Childhood Technical Assistance Center)—
    www.nectac.org
PACER* Center—www.pacer.org
    (*Parent Advocacy Coalition for Educational Rights)
Parent to Parent—USA—www.p2pusa.org
Parent to Parent/Family Support Network of the High Country—
    www.parent2parenthighcountry.org
Parents with Disabilities Online—www.disabledparents.net
Raising Special Kids (AZ)—raisingspecialkids.org
Special Kids Today—www.specialkidstoday.com
Starlight Starbright Children's Foundation—www.starlight.org
Through the Looking Glass—lookingglass.org/index.php

Personal/Technology:

Abilicorp—www.abilicorp.com

AbleNet—www.ablenetinc.com

Adaptations by Adrian—adaptationsbyadrian.com

Aids for Arthritis—www.aidsforarthritis.com

ATIA (Assistive Technology Industry Association)—www.atia.org

Canine Assistants—www.canineassistants.org

Chair Wear by CozyCoats of Vermont—www.cozycoats.com

Eagle Eyes Project—Boston College—www.bc.edu/eagleeyes

Easy Access—www.easyaccessclothing.com

emPOWERing Wheelchair Users—powerwheelchairusers.blogspot.com

Enabling Devices—enablingdevices.com

Fashion Moves—www.fashionmoves.org

Freshette—www.freshette.com

FrogPad—frogpad.com

GimpGear—www.gimpgear.us

Hummingbird Sipper—www.hands-free-drinking.com

Independent You—www.independentyou.com

Mouse Bean—www.mousebean.com/home.htm

NaturalPoint Optical Tracking Systems—www.naturalpoint.com

NECTAC (National Early Childhood Technical Assistance Center)—
www.nectac.org

Simplantex—www.simplantex.co.uk

Special Clothes—www.special-clothes.com

Specially for You, Inc.—www.speciallyforyou.net

USA TechGuide—www.usatechguide.org

WheelchairGear—www.wheelchairgear.com

Play/Recreation:

Accessible parks (listing by state)—www.ncpad.org/parks

adaptivePlay—www.adaptiveplay.org

Beyond Play—www.beyondplay.com

Boundless Playgrounds—www.boundlessplaygrounds.com

(Amy and Peter' Barzach's baby, Jonathan, had SMA; Amy wrote <u>Accidental Courage, Boundless Dreams</u>)

Camp Barnabas—www.campbarnabas.org

(Featured on Extreme Makeover: Home Edition)

Camp Courageous—www.campcourageous.org

Camp Promise-West—www.firstgiving.com/camppromisewest

Camp Sunshine—www.campsunshine.org

Center for Courageous Kids—www.courageouskids.org

Champ Camp—www.champcamp.org

Dragonfly Toy Co.—dragonflytoys.com

emPOWERing Wheelchair Users—powerwheelchairusers.blogspot.com

IKAN Sports Foundation—www.ikansportsfoundation.org

MD Family Fun—www.mdfamilyfun.org

MDA Summer Camp—www.mdausa.org/clinics/camp

Miracle League of the Triangle—www.miracleleagueofthetriangle.com

NCPAD (National Center on Physical Activity and Disability)—
www.ncpad.org

(The) Painted Turtle *(a Hole in the Wall camp)*—
www.thepaintedturtle.org/turtle

Pocket Full of Therapy—www.pfot.com

Power Soccer USA—www.powersoccerusa.net

Preston's H.O.P.E.—www.prestonshope.com

(Preston had SMA)

Shane's Inspiration—www.shanesinspiration.org

Catherine Curry-Williams, Founder/Exec Program Director

(Catherine's son, Shane, had SMA)

Victory Junction Gang—www.victoryjunction.org
Wheelchair Hockey League—www.thewchl.com

'Kitchen-Sink' Resources

CariKelleyTravels—www.ytbtravel.com/carikelley
   (Cari's daughter, Jacquie, has SMA)
Google Alert (SMA and other updates)—www.google.com/alerts
Holy Experience: Ann Voskamp—www.aholyexperience.com
   (Two of Ann's nephews had SMA)
House, M.D.—www.fox.com/house
   (Executive producer/writer Garrett Lerner's son, Zeke, has SMA—benwinship@aol.com)
Joie de Vivre Designs and Fine Gifts—www.jdvdesigns.com
   (Emily's daughter, Aubrey, has SMA)
Larkie Lu Bows—www.larkielubows.com
   (Gina's daughter, Larkie, has SMA and Down syndrome)
Larry's Home Designs—www.larryshomedesigns.com
   (Larry Stauffer and his brother, Stan, have SMA)
Lomonaco Design—www.lomonacodesign.com
   (Nicole, graphic designer, has SMA)
Louise Smith—Lessons of Life—www.TheLessonsofLife.com
   (Louise's niece, Rebecca, has SMA)
(The) Suite Life of Lucy and Ethel—
   thesuitelifeoflucyandethel.blogspot.com
   (Blog by Helen and Cindy Schaefer, mom to Kevin, Type 2. A variety of resources is listed on the blog; in addition, the blog features spotlights on SMA families and others with 'special assignments')
Thought for the Day—www.tftd-online.com

'Threads'

Angel Threads—www.angelthreads.com
Baby Threads—www.babythreads.net
Grannie Threads—www.granniethreads.com
(Jodi's baby, Jordan, had SMA)

If you would like to submit a resource,
please contact me at jeffreyb@skybest.com

A Word (or Two!) of Thanks

We never knew all who rallied around us in some fashion during our Jeffrey journey because of sheer numbers and requested anonymity of many benefactors. We'll also never know how far-reaching the influence of Jeffrey's brief earth visit may continue to be, but we do hope the rippling effects of his special touch continue in some capacity long after we are gone.

Even after twelve years, we extend heartfelt gratitude to our families, friends, neighbors, community churches, and the other earth angels who boosted us in any way, especially those who faithfully included our family in their prayers. In particular, the faculty and staff at Mountain View Elementary School seemed to know what we needed long before we did.

Throughout the years, SMA family members across the world have provided not only names for the special dedication, but enthusiasm and ongoing encouragement for this project. Because of online opportunities ranging from Facebook to Twitter to the blog and groups such as SMASpace, SMA Support, Families of SMA, and SMA Friends, I have had the pleasure of meeting hundreds of 'brothers and sisters' during our Jeffrey journey and look forward to meeting hundreds more!

A very special acknowledgement goes to my folks, (JoAnn and the late Elton Derden), my brother Paul and his family (Jaymie, Jonathan, and Bethany), my mother-in-law (Nell), and extended family for, simply, everything. In addition, two very special pals, Cindy Schaefer, who wrote the foreword and currently shares blogging duties with me, and Ravelle Whitener, who wrote *A Tiny Angel* and designed the original perfect cover (and subsequently inspired some of the current one), deserve kudos for their generous contributions in many capacities.

I'm not sure what we would have done without Gary Barber's compassion. Somehow, he made the worst 'event planning' imaginable—our baby's funeral and burial—manageable. All families needing such services should be so lucky.

Big thankful hugs go to my husband, Randy, for an incredible abundance of patience and understanding and for allowing me to shirk cooking and housecleaning responsibilities on occasion (okay, on MANY occasions) in order to write the original book and the subsequent updates... and now the reissue! The same goes to Matthew and Katie, who became more self-reliant out of necessity during work on the earlier versions and who are now putting what they learned to good use as they venture farther and farther into the realm of independence.

To the many angels who keep watch over us from their heavenly posts on a daily basis—thank you!

Finally, mere words are inadequate in thanking our Heavenly Father for sending Jeffrey, such a glorious surprise, to our family and for holding us upright during our Jeffrey assignment, allowing us to see beyond SMA's devastation to such unexpected wondrous blessings. Consequently, we hope that our actions speak louder than words and are indicative of the revelations that have enhanced our family as we continue this very special journey for the remainder of our earthly time...

A
Special
Dedication

Note About
A Special Dedication

SMA's intense, wicked path of destruction begins with the pronouncement of the diagnosis and prognosis of this killer disease. There is no end. Yet.

It seemed fitting to include a dedication to those whose lives have risen to the challenges of SMA, so I began gathering names and permission to publish them. With relatively minimal effort in the beginning, hundreds of names surfaced, and hundreds have been added on a regular basis since then... until there are now more than a thousand. Hundreds more.

The 'relatively minimal effort' required for the first collection of names quickly graduated to a passion, and some might say it's eased into an obsession. I couldn't disagree.

This simple tribute recognizes a mere handful of those who have somehow paid their dues for involuntary induction into the world of SMA.

Only the first names or initials are listed if I was unable to contact the families and/or procure permission. They are by no means slighted in honor or memory.

Sincere thoughts and prayers are extended to the families of those who earned their wings after this printing and to all newcomers to the family of SMA.

Congratulations to the families and individuals with SMA who demonstrate such tenacity and gusto in life, particularly when they shift the focus to the needs of someone *else*. What an amazing group. An amazing family.

I am proud to be a part of it.

If you would like to add a name to the dedication or make revisions of any kind for future printings, contact me at jeffreyb@skybest.com or P.O. Box 964, Jefferson, NC 28640. Thank you.

Key to specially-marked names:

BVVL—Brown-Vialetto-Van Laere syndrome, a rare motor neuron disease similar to SMA. For more info, visit The Olive Branch Fund—www.theolivebranchfund.org
SMARD—Spinal Muscular Atrophy with Respiratory Distress

A Special Dedication

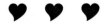

...to honor those living with SMA...

Samantha ('Sami') Abraham * Mariana ('Marianis') Moreano Acevedo *
Makayla ('Kaykay') Adams * Mariah ('Yahyah') Adams *
Rhonda Dee Adkins * 'Aila' * Brooke Alexis-Lynn Akers * Faith Ann Akers *
Gabriella ('Gabby') Marie Aleman * Crystal Allbritton * Mar Álvarez *
Victor Alvarez * Miles ('Sunshine' / 'Buddy Boy') Ambridge *
Samantha ('Sam') Marie Amend * Suzanne LaPrise Ammons *
Roman Walker Anderson * Isabella Andrade * Bradly Alan Andrews *
Malena Angelini * Mallory Armbrustmacher * Devin Tyler Arnold *
Rosana Arteta * Anita (Amy) Ashdon * Amanda Ashton *
Iceis Danielle Augustino * Laura Janice Bairett *
Jensen Elizabeth Victoria Baldwin * Lauren Ball *
Emma ('M&M') Mary Banach * Nikki Barker * Alexis Barr *
Karah Elyse Barry * Julia Maria Bartczak * Joseph ('Jojo') Brady Baudin *
Angela ('Angie') Bebee-Wright * Sawyer Beechler * Laura ('Lala') Begic *
Samuel Bell * Carlos Emanuelle Benejam * Kelsey L. Bergbigler *
Carson Andrew Berry * Cooper Anderson Berry * Lisa Bertolini *
Grace ('Gracie') Elizabeth Bertram * Lauren Marie Biancucci *
Mary Kate Bigelow * Christian Bilbay *
Alexander ('Alex') Gabriel Billerman *
Victoria ('Tori') Rose Billerman * Aschdon Lorenz Birkle *
Chessa Rose Marko Birrell * Larkin ('Larkie') Bish *
Morgan ('Yady') Riley Bishop * Alex Blair * Lielén ('Lee') Blasini *
Halsey Blocher * Krista Bodzo * Jenna ('JJ') Boguhn * Jerika Bolen *
Alex Bolton * Eleanor Bolton * Jack Bolton * Sam Bolton*
Ryan Cooper Bonsett * Jerry Book * Jennifer Bordelon *

Sarah Borowski * John J. Bottone, IV * Evan Breton *
Patricia May Bristow * Michael Brodsky * Greg Brooker *
Trevor James ('TJ') Broton * Caitlin ('Caitie' / 'Cait') Brown *
Maxwell Brown * Ryan Andrew Brown * Samantha A. Brown *
Ashley Bruner * Dwight ('Buddy') Bryan * Adyn Kassidy Bucher *
Dustin James Bucholtz * Aiden Scott Bundy * Kelly Buonaccorsi *
Joanna Emma Buoniconti * Logan ('Logie') Bailey Burch *
Jane E. Burdette * Samuel Burnett * Dwayne Burrwell * Chloe Bush *
Garrett ('GB') Allen Buthe * Kyle Donovan Byrd *
Lauren Chelsea Byrd * Pranav C. * Brianna Mariah Cagle *
Shelly Rachel Cahlon * Michael (Owen) Cain *
Hayden Christine Calafiore * Adam Calderwood *
Corinna Elizabeth Calise * Roberto Camiro *
Tambryn Ember Campbell * Isabel Michelle Campos *
Courtney Paige Canfield * Falon C. * Alba Blasco Carbonell *
Mary (Beth) Carollo * 'Carolyn' * Jamey Carrington *
Christopher Cassel * Alyssa Castagna * Crystal Cevallos * Li-lee Cha *
Malachi Chapman * Jocelyn Chen * Kalei ('Toot') Danae Chisholm *
Josy Chow * Ella Christopher * MayMay Chun * Jerry W. Clark *
Lucile Clavier * Kenneth Lloyd ('K.L.') Cleeton II * Mary Cobley *
Lindsay Kaitlynn Cochran * Emily Nicole Coddington *
Jane Coggins * Jonas Coleman * Ta'Bria Neosha Collier *
Brianna Connelly * Veronique Conner * Kristen Connors *
Jimmy Contento * Amadaya Cooke * Holly Cooper * Malik A. Cosby *
Kerri Costello * Ryan Cottor * Rebeckah ('Beckah') Courdt *
Carrie Cowgill * Julia ('J-Girl') Swan Cramer * Sydney C. *
Kristina Creekmore * Andrew R. Creighton * Miranda Cremeens *
Neil Crosswaite * Katelyn ('Katerbug') Rose Crowder * Blanche Cuba *
Joshua Cueter * Dylan Jack Cuevas * Jada Cusick * Selena Cusick *
Jeremy Dack * McKenzie L. Damon * Khalil Dana *
Alexandria ('Alex') Hope Darce * Jo D'Archangelis *
Jonathon Meyers Davies * Casey Wayne Daws * Alexa Dectis *

246

Isabella Del Campo * Connor DeLuca * Jack DeRooy-Harris *
Pierina Naori Miyadi Diaz * Ariana Leigh Dindzans *
Ares Jun su Dobson * Samantha Giovanna Dodaro *
Sophia ('Pumpkin') Karin Doebbert *
Sydney ('C-Bug') Madison Landry Donovan *
Kaylee ('KiKi') Shae Dorfman * Michael (Gray) Dougherty *
Debbie Drake * Drew John Drazenovich * Morgan Duffy *
Charlene Dumont * Kaige ('Kaigers') James Russell Dunham *
Brendon Dupree * Alexandria Dzimitowicz * Amanda Eads *
Cody Edwards * Hunter Edwards * Natalie Edwards *
Daniel ('Danny') Egan * Skylar ('Sky') Eichele * Hanna Eide *
Nisar Elahi * Anita ('Anix') Eleonora * Taylor Renee Ellington *
Austin Michael Elliott * Peyton ('Beauty Girl' / 'Pey') Lola Elsner *
Tyler Engel * Colin Joseph English * Jaxon Jeremy English *
Tabitha Michelle English * Greyson Shepherd Erwin *
Cassandra Victoria Evans * Ruth Everard * Kindal Patricia Evers *
Sierra ('C. C.') Journey Factor * Maxime Paul Famin * Ray Fantel *
Fionna Faroon * Aileen L. Farrell * Alexa ('Seccy') Caitlyn Felix *
Héctor Álvarez Fernández * Cole Kaycee Fiedler * Alexis Fifelski *
Leah Finch * Sam Fisher * Shira ('Little Miss Boops') Fisher *
Austin Blayne Fitch * Henrik Fjelde * Jon Fleming *
Joshua Joel Fletcher * Racquel Flores * Barry Lee Fodor *
Cindy Ann Fodor * Howard H. Y. Fok * Kaleb Folbrecht *
Edmond Fordham, II * Ashley Lynn Fox * Malorie Alexis Fox *
Bernadette Francois * Jennifer Franey * Matthew Franey *
Eve ('Evie') Darian Frederick * Jack Freedman *
Haley ('Boo Boo') Brianna Freeman * Lauryn Freundl *
Haley Frieler * Morgan Rose Fritz * Emily Rose Gallagher *
Thomas Gallagher * Leanne M. Gallipeau *
Alivianna ('Ali') Brighid Gallup * Montse Font Garcia *
Zachary Gardner * Addison ('Addy') Grace Garner * Janna Gates *
Jennifer Gaudreau * Sophia ('Pooka') B. Gaynor * Jack Gellner *

Amira Lilliana Sky George * Arturo Charles George *
Lauren Elizabeth Geraghty * Claire Gibbs * Lauren Gibbs *
Zachary Aaron Gilbert * 'Giorgos' * Tom Giumelli *
Melissa Jane Gleason * Christopher Golden * Elisa Golden *
Emma Hope Goldsberry * Austin Goluba * Nora Madison Gooden *
Jacob Christopher Goodson * Zoe Graffam * Christie Grande *
Bailey Grant * Aubrey Jeanne-Marie Green * Sara Rose Greene *
Ryan Gregory * Zoe Grisez * Tanner ('TanMan') Grover *
Suellen Groves * Kyle Gundy * Nicholas Gustafson * Yvette Haas *
Elizabeth Lee Hallam * Ragnar Emil Hallgrimsson *
Destiny ('Dezi') Hamilton * Hugo Hammarin *
Lanie Elizabeth Hannah * Kaitlyn Harapchuk * Mackinley Hardison *
Michaella ('Micah') Gene Cysouw Hargrave * John Harris *
Abbey Lee Hassel * Garrett Steven Hassel * Kaitlyn Hatchard *
Karl Hatt * Douglas ('Doug') Hayes * Kameron ('Kam') M. Hayes *
Mark D. Healy * Ann Heathcote * Silvana Helliwell *
Kaelan Bradlee Henry * Karlie Miya Henry * Nathan Herman *
Tyler Hernandez * Jessica Elizabeth Hetzel * Patrick Higgins *
David Hile * Richard F. Hill, II * Sunni-Louise ('Sunni-Lou') Hind *
Videl Skye Hinke * Shelby Hintze * Ashley Hodges *
Jaclyn ('Jackie') Quinn Hoffmann * 'Hol' * Connor Holdsworth *
Julian Lavelle Holman * Sydney Alyse Horak *
Evelyn ('Evie') Horton * Lexx Michael Howell * Dave Hughes *
Mia Danielle Hultgen * William Huntley * Joshua ('Baby J') Hurd *
Taryn Barbara Hussey * Oliver Philip Huston * Linh Thi Huynh *
Quoc David Huynh * Haylee ('Miss Anne' / 'Hayleekins') Hynes *
Reagan Imhoff * Alexa ('Dumplin') Ivey * Meg J ('MJ') * Lisa Jahn *
Cooper M. James * Chloe ('Peanut') Ann Jamieson *
Ludmila Javurková * Isaac Jessee * Brandon James Johnson *
Jami Johnson * Landon ('Mister Wister') Robert Johnson *
Owen Johnson * Reilly Blake Johnson *
Charley ('Chazza') Marie Johnston *

Kazi ('Kamakazi') Mark Johnston * Christopher Jones *
Dana ('My Smiley Girl') Lynn Jones *
Daniel ('My Handsome Guy') Thomas Jones * Dayton A. Jones *
John L. Jones, II * Vivianne Heather Jones * 'Juana' *
Austin Riley Jumper * Vicki Lynn Jurney-Taylor * Corinne Kagan *
Kasey Kaler * Jennifer ('Jen') Kariman * Keanu Kauwe *
Julia Katherine Kay * Melanie Keefer * Christoph Keller *
Jacqueline ('Jacquie') Marie Kelley * Michael Kelley *
Morgan ('Princess Morgan') Joyce Kelly * Brielle G. Kennedy *
Brooke A. Kennedy * Allison P. Kerns * Heather Kerstetter *
Allegra ('Leggy') Keys * Che Hun Kim * Heather Kimes *
Allison Renea King * Bradley (Austyn) King * Easton E. King *
Brett Kingsley * Nicole Kinzel * Kelly Kirchstein * Kyle Kirk *
Megan Kirk * Ingrid Klein * Derk Kok * Ron Kort * Jack Kotheimer *
Alyssa Kotsopoulos * Christel Alexina Kotte * Ewa Kozak *
Allyson ('Angel Ally') Krajewski * Alyssa Krider *
Bella Ksontini * Addison ('Addy') Kuester * Brian Kupferschmidt *
Holly M. Kupferschmidt * Victoria ('Tori') Lacey *
Daniel Marc Lajoie * Jessica Faith Lamb * Scarlett Rose Landefeld *
Anna Landre * Taysen ('Taye-Taye') Langstraat * Tonje Larsen *
Peter Laudan * Michelle Laverdiere * Emily Hope Lee *
Jocelyn Paige Lee * Jessica Lehman * Angeles Aracely Leon *
Zeke Lerner * Shaun Michael Lesniak * Adora Brooke Lewis *
Antonio Eric Lewis * Ian Paul Lewis * Satori Lewis *
Sierra Rae Lewis * Matt Liegel * Tommy Lim * Julia Lincoln *
Jack Thomas Lindaman * Justin Linn * Jamie Lino * Troy Lino *
Gabriella ('Gabbie') Rose Lisacchi * Brynlee Belle Liston *
AnMei Liu * Emma Ruth Lockwood * Nicholas James Lockwood *
Charlotte Florence Lohner * Nicole Lomonaco * Caitlin Long *
Jackson ('Jack') Long * Carlos ('GTA Charlie') López * Ian Lopez *
Samantha Lorey * Benjamin Lou * Dakin Lovelace (SMARD) *
Summer Luke * Llarell Alejandro Hernández Luna *

Sofia Anne-Marie Lynsdale * Jeffrey Macak *
Hayden Phillip MacIntyre * Taylin Amily Mackay * 'Maddalena' *
Vivianna Madera * Bryce Madsen * Tara Ann Mahoney *
Jennifer Malatesta * Carolyn Malloy * Brooke Ashley Malone *
Ryan Maly * Austin Alan Manning * Linda Napolitano Manning *
Cody Mannion * Ryan ('Ryno') Matthew Manriquez *
Ariyana ('Nanna Bug') Marcel * Rachel Markley *
Karen Gaseni Marlow * Amy M. Marquez *
Jesus ('Chuy') Alexandro Marquez-Harper *
Alexander ('Alex') Marshall * Micah ('Moocher') Paul Marshall *
Alexandria Martin * 'Martin' * Shawn Martin *
Elena Gomez Martinez * William Thomas Mason * Lori Matthews *
Yuliya Matyushenko * Jonathan Maul * Danae Maxwell *
Preston Maxwell * Shayla Maxwell * Danielle Maycox * Nathan Mayer *
Courtney Jeanne Mazzella * Skyler McAdams *
Mark ('Marco') McCarthy * Melissa ('Mo') McCreary *
Emily Jean McCulley * Brianna McDanel *
Natalie ('Little Bear') Christina McDonald *
Rachael Marie McDonald * Kiley McDonnell * Patrick McDonnell *
Taylor McDonnell * Aaron J. McGirt * Daniel Joseph McHale *
Jillian McIntosh * Bernie McKeough * Tierney Lee McKown *
Fred McLees * Ava McLin * Deirdre ('Deedee') Medina *
Shane Megale * Brandon ('Brando') David Meinke * Isabella Melara *
Hayron Mérida Friman * Madisyn ('Madi') Alon Mevissen *
Marianne Middlebrook * Kennedy Migchelbrink *
Anna ('Souslik') Migrina * Inés Bravo Miguel *
Melissa Anne Milinovich * Aleena Hope Miller * Alyssa Miller *
Bruce Michael Miller * Jenica Mae Miller * Kalei Ann Miller *
Katelyn Jeaneane Miller * Leah ('Beantsy') Jean Miller *
Katie Mirabile * Haley Christiana Mitchell * Annah Nikole Mobus *
Rev. Richard A. Moe * Mary Elizabeth Montague *
Joshua ('Josh') Monteiro *

LeAnna ('Princess LeAnna' / 'Anna Banana') Reneé Moore *
Ben Morris * Jon Morrow * Lindsay Marie Muench *
Vivien ('Fish') Mullett *(sister to Rebecca Mullet & aunt to Ruby Gilbury)* *
Destiny A. Muniz * Austin Emerson Munro * Erin S.A. Murakami *
Garrison Murph * Connor Murphy * Eric Murphy *
Michael P. Murphy * Maryann Musselman *
Lindsey Renee Muszkiewicz * Joseph Michael Myckaniuk *
Preben Myhre * Pratyush Nalam * Kim Napiwocki * Thomas Narum *
Lilyán Navarro * Syeda Shagufta ('Shaguf') Naz * Laura Nellen *
Ben Nelson * Brady Nelson * Colby Nelson * Grace Nelson *
Jodi Nelson (& Juni, service dog!) * Mary Grace Nelson *
Kaitlyn Nguyen * Paige Caroline Nixon * Johnny Noblett *
Daniela Noboa * Tyshan ('Ty') Malic Norman * Mikaela Rose Norris *
Mariella Norris-Garcia * Dianne Pollie Nuell * Karen Maree O'Brien *
Shannon O'Brien * Ethan James Och *
Chelsea ('Sweet Pea') Bleu O'Donnell * Christopher Ogden *
Riley Ogden * Amelia O'Hare * Conor ('Ginger') O'Kane *
Austin Olander * Jeffrey Olander * Jonathan G. Olivares *
John Olson * Shane Oltmans * Casey Eugene O'Neill *
Colin Robert O'Neill * Jennifer Onsum * Steve Onsum *
Gayle Ortega * Julia Marie Ortego * Pamela M. Ortego *
Peggy Sue MacKenzie Overbey * Melynnda Overholtz *
Alaysha Álvarez Pagán * Hunter Christian Pageau (SMARD) *
Irina ('Ira') Parfionova * Cheyenne Parra * Madison Parrotta *
Jack William Parry * Tori Nicole ('T. Cole') Partee *
Kaitlyn Debra Johanna Pas * Marina Paskina *
Charles (Logan) Patrick * John ('Chef John') Pawula * Holly Payne *
Katherine Pecora * Aul Pedajas * Thomas ('Tommy') Hart Pence *
Kimberley Pendergrass * Camie Perez * Ameila Rose Perry *
Autumn Kay Persinger * Michael ('Mikey') Pezzuto *
Aaron David Phelps * Jay Pierce Phillips * Nicholas ('Nick') Piazza *
Morgan Pierce * Danielle ('Meimei'- sister) Seah Xin Ping *

Paolo ('Underrunner') Pisano * Avery ('Miss Beautiful') Pitzen *
Robyn Marie Plaster * Mark Plocharczyk * Chaz Podolnick *
Patie Polczyk * Tyler Pollock * Isaac Reed Postma *
Sydney Grace Potjer * Vita Potocnik * Steven Nicholas Potter *
LaMondre Pough * Kelli Prather * Aidan Vaughn Press *
Gerrit Ivan Pretorius * Colby Pretz * Hannah Nicole Price *
Maya Pringle * Danielle ('Dani') Pruitt * David Gregory Pruitt *
Cole Pulkrabek * Margaret ('MJ') Purk * Zachary Peyton Pylychuk *
Caiden Lee Pynenberg * Augusto Maria Quatrini *
Natalie Marie Quintana * Sam Rader * Caitlyn Eleanor Radocy *
Jacqueline Radtke * Jessica Radtke * Logan P. Ragland *
Peter Jerry Ramirez * Jasmine Rankin * Noel Ratapu * Venla Raty *
Elizabeth A. Raymond * Nicholas J. Raymond, IV * Madison Rose Reed *
Connor William Reilly * Pamela ('Pam') Patricia Renshaw *
Camilita Reyes * Ava-Isabel Kekaimalie Rezentes * Sam Rice *
Kelly Richardson * Melissa Richardson * Brett Richter *
Karson Michael Riggs * Kathy Riley * 'Riley' * Vincenzo ('Vinny') Rini *
Shanice Robertson * Trevor Allen Robinett * Izzabella ('Bella') Rodgers *
Alexa Rodriguez * Gerardo ('Jerry') Rodriguez, Jr. * Nuris Rodriguez *
Brian C. Ronningen * Courtney Brooke Rosas * Ross Cory Rosenfeld *
Bernie Ross * Ana Marcela ('Marcy') Rubio * Charles (Cosmo) Rudd *
Cael Charles Rudkin * Karlson Russell Ruhle *
Minouche Manon Ruiz * John ('Jay') Runkle * Savanna Rush *
Lindsay Marie Russell * Nathan Edward Russell *
Thomas Daniel Russell * Jacqueline S. * Joshua S. * Sébastien St-Jean *
Veronica Rose St. Onge * Jesana Saksi * Marisol Saksi * Cory Saldana *
Katherine ('Kate') Saldana * Kayla M. Samz *
Destiny ('Princess') Hope Sanchez * Brooklynn Rae Santos *
Jackson Saville * Samuel Thomas Sawyer * Jake Saxton *
Brittany Jean Saylor * Kendra Nicole Scalia * Kevin William Schaefer *
Nicole ('Nicci') Schauerte * Samuel Schoenborn * Sarah J. Schwegel *
Anna Rose Scurria * Joshua Scurria * Sara Mackenzie Seavers *

Steven Bret Sebastianelli * Rayanna Jane Seffens * Kavya Sehgal *
Alexander Ayres Sequeira * Ashley Elizabeth Sequeira * Olena Sh *
Brandon Shaffer * Sohum Shah * Brandon Jacob Shaklee *
Gunn Aas Shaw * Charlotte Sherwood *
Maddison ('Maddi') Elise Ronnie Sherwood (SMARD) *
Brooke Shetler * Kale Robert Shiesley * Emma Grace Shifflett *
Thomas Shindle * Maia Shockley * Nolan Ostin Shofner *
Bama ('Jam-Jam') Davis Shore * Isabella ('Izzy') Maria Sicoli *
Morgan James Sidor * Abraham Silva *
Maliylah ('Lil Miss') Imani Silva * Arya Channeng Singh *
Andy Sinish * Regan Dean Sink * Andrew Slay and his 'Buddies' *
Jacob Cole Slaymaker * Sarah Jane Smallpiece *
Courtney Lynn Smith * Deanna Smith * Joanne ('Joie') Smith *
Joseph Bennett Smith * Kristen Smith * Madison Smith *
Riley ('Smiley Riley') Smith * Roswitha (Anne) Smith *
Sheila Smith * Kyla Snelling * Laurie Sore * Hannah Soyer *
William ('Billy') George Spiegel, Jr. * Susan Pedersen Spingler *
Ethan ('E-Man') Isaac Spivey * Jake Stamper * Larry Stauffer *
Stan Stauffer * Lynn Otterness Stern * Amber Kristin Stewart *
Lynsey Stewart * Kristen ('Little Girl') Still * William Stocker *
Whitnee Lana Stoddard * Charles Stopford * Paige ('PJs') Jayden Stout *
Gwendolyn DeBard Strong * Philip J. Struble * Skylar Swanson *
Danny Sweetman * Michael Sweetman *
Helen Elizabeth ('Betsy') Neel Swetnam *
Katherine ('Katie') Kirby Swetnam * Addison ('Addi') Swims *
Charles ('Charlie') Robert Sykora * Joseph Szumigalski *
Angelo Szychowski * Ethan ('Mommy's Little Chicken') William Takacs *
William Tamiso * Elizabeth ('Lizzie') Tanner * Patrick G. Tansey, Jr. *
Alonso Gabriel Tapia * Mandy Lucieal Tawn * Alex Telenson *
Alana R. Theriault * Jade Hailey Theriault * Kyle Thomas *
Rhylee Thompson (SMARD) * Meredith Tokar * Franca Tomasella *
Julio Chojeda Torres * Leopoldo ('Leo') Anthony Tortora *

253

Hannah Michelle Rose Trail * Ayden Dale Trammell *
Haydon Travers * Gina Trotto * Adri Truter * Farzana ('Faca') Tsabita *
Apollonia Tsanta * Radmila Turanjanin * Stella Turnbull * Sam Turner *
John Leslie Tuss * Arynn Tyrrell * Ezamudin ('Ezam') Umat *
Far'ain ('Paah') Umat * Gazlia ('Lia') Umat * Amy Urbanski *
Marco ('Tesoro'—*treasure*) Antonio Valverde, Jr. * Holli VanderWyk *
Kayla Grace Vanderzanden * Rebecca ('Bex') Grace Van Fraassen *
Jacqueline ('Jackie') Van Herk-Kennedy * Babbe Vanneste *
Lia Renee Cobos Varela * Flor Maria Vargas * Matthew Varney *
Amanda Velez * Lisa Velez * Kennady J. Verbsky * Steven Verdile *
Madison ('Maddy') Alexandra Versuk * Ryan ('Ry') Christopher Viano *
Serenne Vikeboe * Madison ('Madi') Villegas * Leah Vogedes *
Bentley Jo Vondrak * Jaycie Rene Vondrak * Kennedi Marie Vondrak *
Peter Voskovitch * Patricia ('Pat') Agnes Walden * Taylor Rae Wallace *
Matthew Avery Wallis * Kerry Nicole Walsh * Jacob Waltier *
Matthew Warren * Callie Mae Watkins * Blake Watson * Matt Watson *
Cubby Wax * Christopher Bruce Weber * Evan David Weise (SMARD) *
Tessa Marie Weisenberger * Lyza Jane Weisman * Kelly Webb Werdin *
Olivia Werstein (and BFF, Erinne Rose Williams) *
Dinand van Werven * William (Tyler) Wester * Karen Wheeler *
Sean Patrick Wheeler * Peter R. Whitaker * Ryan Michael White *
Gideon ('Gus') Dalton Whittamore * Essie Whitteker *
Erinne Rose Williams (and BFF, Olivia Werstein) *
Sacha Monet Williams * Jessica Willis * Terry Willoughby *
Todd Alexander Willoughby * Alexis Marie Wilson * Brett Jacob Wilson *
Bryce David Wilson * Gidget Kerrington Winward *
Nikolas John Winward * Margrett ('Meg') Witkowski *
Martin Witkowski * Madison Wolff * Alvy Wong * Elizabeth Ann Wood *
Melissa ('Lisa') A. Woods * Adam David Woodson *
Jessica ('Fusser') Joy Wosika * Bethany R. Wright * Carmen Yau *
Victoria Yenzer * Jonathan Tiong Soon Yi * James ('Jay') Allen Young *
Lucy Jean Zahn * Stacy Lee Zoern

...to remember those who have earned their wings...

Deirdre Ann Abraldes * Trinity ('Petunia') Elizabeth Aguilar *
Lindsay Suzanne Alexander * Eric Harrison Alford *
Dustyn ('Doo-nut') Edward Boyd Amaral-Hicks *
Benjamin ('Benjimano') M. Amiss * 'Amy Sue' *
Isabella ('Bella') Ann Anderson * Kyleigh Mae Anhorn *
Ami Ankilewitz * Kathryn Rose Anthony * Sofia Victoria Aracena *
Nicki Allison Ard (Miss Wheelchair America 2001) *
James ('Jaime') Thomas Armstrong * Tracy Lynn Armstrong *
Henry ('Hank') Anthony Ashdon, Jr. * Tonna Louise Winter Ashdon *
Mary Jane ('My Lady Jane') Tesch Ausse *
Hailey ('Sugar Bear') Michelle Aversman * Jordan Azar *
Lauren Miah Azar * 'Baby Angel' * Sean Christopher Bacon *
Skylar William Bahrenburg * Beth Bailey * Jeffrey Thomas Baldwin *
Zoey ('Baby Zoey') Lee Banschbach-Russ * Bella Mia Barberena *
Callum Anthony Barker * Neil ('Little Neil') Barker * Lily Barnett *
Nathan Barnett * Colten Michael Barnicle * Jonathan Peter Barzach *
Bentley ('Boo') Bassamore * Luigi Estevao Batirola *
Emmy Rose Baugher * Jennifer Marie Beachnau * Eli Beasley-Wright *
Courtney Elyse Beauchesne * Tylah Millicent Bell *
Jeanette Avery Benejam * Justin ('Bubba') Wyatt Berge *
Richard ('Rik')Lynn Berkenpas * Martina Paz Berlin *Jacob Berrier *
Milla Charlette Bevis * Ruby Bianchi-Hobbs *
Brooke ('Pumpkin') Leigh Binning * Maggie Wyn Bonesteel *
Matthew C. Bonnell * Lily Emma Boots *
Lainie ('Lou Lou') Grace Border * Taylor Kate Bowser *
Joseph Paul Box * Paul Joseph Box * Marcello Brandao *

Landyn Edward Dean Breiner * Allie ('Baby Allie') Brenner *
Mitchell ('Baby M') John Briggs * Barbara Ann Bristow *
Kinsey Bronston * Makalia Renee Brown *
Tiffany ('Tiff') Marquis Brown * Seán James Browne-Keating *
Johnathan Boyd Browning * Montanna ('Monty') Jean Brownlaw *
Zarlee Rose Brownlaw * Jonathan Brunetti *
Kelsey ('Kelsemanneke') Bruynseels * Kyle Raymond Bry *
Michelle Buchman * Emma B. * Celia Lolly Bultemeyer *
Annabelle ('Belle Boo') Rose Burfitt * Madison Burger *
Ethan Burnett * Grant William Burns * Owen Michaelis Burns *
Andrew ('Andy') Glenn Butler * Caleb William Butler *
Mark S. Butler * Audra Claire Caine * Felipe Thadeu Antunes Calegari *
Kelsey Campagna * Braden ('Tumbleweed') Ray Campbell *
Hannah Jean Campbell * Alex Camwell *
Michael ('Mikey') Anthony James Capper * Ian ('Buggaboo') Carleton *
Alex Michael Raymond Carter * Daniel ('Danny Boy') Cevallos *
Maddox William Nasedo Chance * Ms. Ngai Kit Ching *
Ke'aja Tiaris Chisholm * Ilsa Mae Chowaniec * Ashley Christianson *
Penny Louann Claar * Kendra Michelle Clark * Michael Keith Clark *
Nicholas Roman Clark * Riley London Clark * Saria Wynelle Clark *
Taylor Michelle Clark * Vickie Lynn Clark *
Grace ('Sunshine') Dyan Coggin * Belle Colchester-Hall *
Curtis ('Curty') Chandler Cole * Mary ('Pooh') Coletti *
Riley Shawn Comeau ('Brother Bear' to Brie & Matti, SMA-free) *
Lilly Robyn Conlan * Tiernan James Conner-Park *
Colin Matthew Connor * Kalani Akiaten Connoy *
Beau ('Chooker') Coogan * Tahj Akeem Cooke * R.J. Corradino *
Taylor Chase Costa * Charlie ('Charlie Bear') J. Cowan * Grant Craig *
Lindsay Craig * Tina Creed * Ashley C. Creighton *
Gavin Patrick Crews * Phoenix Lee ('Our Cheeky Monkey!') Crocker *
Danella ('Danie') Cruz * Shane Alexander Curry-Williams *
Peter Dack * Samir Abbas Dahouk * Ava Grace Dancel-Paguio *

Madison Kate Darlington * Valerie Rose ('Rosie') Davies *
Adam Michael Davis * Fernando De Andrade, Jr. *
Karsten Anne de Boer * Kristin DeBonee * William Defendiefer *
Jessica Mary DeLong * Sophia ('Sophie') Marie Denk * Rebecca Diels *
Emily Laura Domzalski * Michael ('Our Little Man') E. Doyle, Jr. *
Gracie Duke * Ashley Elizabeth Dukes * Kendall Elizabeth Dukes *
Kelly ('Baby Girl') Grace Durham * Brody Durocher *
Connor Mathew Dykman * Justin Cameron Dykman *
Douglas Sawyer Eberhardt * Amy Catherine Edgerton *
Bethan Louise Edwards * Warren Edwards * Jaecob Allen Eggerud *
Taleah Louise English * Samuel ('Sam') Robert Stirling Everard *
Lewis ('Looby Loo') James Farmer * Hannah Grace Fehn *
Jessica Irene Fernandes * Darcy Field *
Andrew ('Booper') Richard Fimbel * Herman Fischer *
Preston Trask Fisher * Mason Alexander Fleck * Shannon Fogard *
Courtney Erin Foley * Eden Kathleen Foley * Bridget Raylene Forstall *
Maranda Rose Forstall * Heather Dawn Frazee * Jacob Ryan Frazee *
Payton James Freeman * Isabella Brynn Freilicher * Bill Freiwald, Jr. *
Lauren Furr * Rhiana Gallagher * Gabriela Guerrero García *
Kathryn ('Katie') Louise Gardner * Dallyce Joy ('DJ') Gartner *
Adrianne ('Sis') Elaine Gayman * Nicoletta Maria Genna *
Alison George * Malia Simone George * Lucia Ana Gerden *
Alejandra Gervais * Jordyn Theresa Gianessi * Hampton Clyde Gilbert *
Ruby Elizabeth Gilbury (niece to Vivien & Rebecca Mullet) *
Christian James Gillen * James Patrick Giroir * Emma Glander *
Kaylie Elizabeth Goddard * Brookes Gordon * Joshua Gordon *
Bryan James Gould * Serena Autumn Graham * Connor Edward Green *
Daniel Green * Emily Norma Green * Marissa Rose Green *
Brittany Leigh Griffin * Patrick Timothy Griffin *
Charlotte ('Char Bar') Elizabeth Grillo * Marley Ann Guay *
Mark Jacob Guilfoile * Matthew Guinta * Jamie Olivia Haapalainen *
Jacob ('Jake') David Haenel *

Cain ('Mommy's Little Soldier') Peter Halstead *
Britta Elise Halvorson * Connor T. Haney * Thomas C. Haney *
Lucas Stephen Hannigan * Dustin James Hanson * Mia Jasmin Haq *
Logan ('Logibear') James Harman * Nikki Renee Harms *
Amanda Kate Harris * Mikayla Grace Harris *
Misti Rose Packlaian Harris * Gavin Michael Harvey *
Shania Jo Hasselman * Ryan Michael Hawn * Miss Wong Wan Hei *
Nicole M. Heimann * Claire Altman Heine * Taija Heinonen *
Mitchel Daniel Henneberry-Robar * Aimee Hernandez *
Sarah Martínez Hernández * Korbin Blaine Hicks *
Ravyn Cae'lynn Hill * Mitchel ('Peanut-Boy') L.R. Hirsch *
Chelsea Hogan * Jacob Blake Holden * Katie Ann Holland *
Jack Buckley Hoogstraten * Andrew Craig Hooker *
Daniel Ryan Howard * June Marie Howsden *
Colten ('Squishy') Hughart * Daniel Blake Humphrey *
Lorraine Frances Humphrey * Ally Cadence Humphries *
Miss Dao Thuy Huong * Brook Taylor Hurst *
Jumaana ('The Silver Pearl') Ibrahima * Bethany Ann Irvine *
Cody Michael Irvine * River ('Rivie') Sky Isherwood * Jonathan Jaffe *
Jet James * Scott ('Pooder') David Jarrett *
Joseph ('Baby Joseph') Bradford Jean *
Autumn ('Bright Eyes') Rose Marie Jeffery * Tristan Edward Jentzsch *
Amy Lynn Jerome * John Xhedrick * Jacob Andrew Johnson *
Miranda ('Randa Panda') Elaine Johnson * Audrey Lynn Jones *
Bronwyn Kate Jones * Christopher ('CJ') Matthew Jones *
Duncan McArthur Jones * Connor Landon Jumper *
David Stephen Jurkovich * Michelle Faye Justice * Ms. Lai Kan *
Kala'i Kauwe * Madisyn ('Madi lu') McGee Kemp *
Lilian ('Lily') Eileen Kennedy * Molly Louise Kennedy *
Emma Lauryn Kindig * Connor King * Denise Renea King *
Jeanetta Louise King * Jamee Lynne Kinney * Shawn Edmund Kinney *
Ava Mae Kloiber * Emersyn Paige Klomp (Emersyn—*Home Strength*) *

Ciara Koo * Liam Koopman * Colin Michael Koos *
Ruth Goldie Krane * Nathaniel Matthew Kroes * Tyler Reginald Kroes *
Alexander ('Alex') Terence Lack * Madelyn Elizabeth Lake *
Aidan Thomas Lay * Elijah ('Eli') Laymance * Linnea Grace Lee *
Reilly ('Our Little Man') Cash Lehman * Jenica Ho Leong *
Alexander Kosta Lipinski * Michael Joseph Lockyer *
Abigail ('Abby') Lynn Loebach * Ronald ('Ronnie') L. Love, II *
Zane ('Zane-e-man') Anthony Carson Love *
Georgia ('Georgie') Lily Lucas * Jordan Lybrand *
Samuel George Lynsdale * Aydan ('Sunshine') Emmanuel Mabe *
Andrea Macak * Daniel Macak * Phillip Macak * Robert Macak *
Jennifer Lorraine Macaulay * Andrew Michael Macbeth *
David Daniel Macbeth * Stephen Macbeth *
Bretton ('Angel Baby') Scott MacLeod * Bharat Maddala *
Luke ('Lukie') Anthony Joseph Maida * Leif Graham Maki *
Casey Lynn Mako * Dylan Stephen Mako * Ivy Lynn Mako *
Marissa Kay Manning * Hodges Chip Manross *
William (Jacobsen) Manross *
Lorelei ('Sweet Pea'/'Pumpkin Eater'/'Boo Bug') Lea Marks *
Jay R. Marlow * John Patrick ('J.P.') Marr-Sisan *
Hannah Morgan Marshall * Logan ('Logie') Wade Martin *
Baylee Mason * Porter Mason * Szel Mason *
Michael Anthony Masterson * Jakob Oliver ('Ollie') Mastin *
Paul Matthews * Stasha Maxwell * Christian Nicholas May *
Callum James ('C. J.') Mccarthy * Sarah Ann McColl *
Kaylee Sue McCorkle * Larissa Jean McCorkle *
Patrick Rowan George McCrone * Mary Kate McDonnell *
Thomas Patrick McDonnell * Justin A. McGirt *
Jack Christopher McKee * Nathan James McKenzie *
Nancy Ellen McLallen * Sondra Lee McLallen * Emily Paige McNabb *
Makayla McPherson * Parker Ray McVay *
Archie Oliver Michel-Malet * Chrystal Marie Miller *

Dace Jade Miller * Kason J. Miller * Swade Jace Miller *
Alyssa Lynne Milliken * Sarah Louise Cook Mills * Austin Gray Minton *
Jewel Essence Mitchell * Shreya Moholkar * Blake James Molloy *
Levi Aron Mooibroek * Ali ('Ali Bugs') Maelaine Marie Moore *
Erick ('Bubbles') Dean Moore * Ramon Arturo Morado, III *
Jacob ('Jake') Lee Morrow * Morgan Sydney Mosby *
Steven Leighton Moyer *
Rebecca Mullett *(sister to Vivien Mullet & aunt to Ruby Gilbury)* *
Cecilia Lehan Murphy * Cianan De Weer Murphy * Paige Louise Myers *
Kalair Mariana Myrick * Doris Navaro * Andrew Evan Neely *
Abigail Negrin * Aaron Blake Nethercutt * Laura Neville *
Timothy (Chance) New * Brian Robert Nicholls * Janet Nicklaus *
Ryan James Nolan * Ryan Thomas Nolan * Brecken Danrek Novotny *
StephanyJo ('Jo Jo') Ann Noyce * Aiden Tomkins Odell *
Rhine Andrew Oliver * Nadia Paola Portillo Olmedo *
Quinn Leslie Graham Scholl Orchard * Jessa Arianna Orr *
Holly Ann Ortego * Leo Ruddick Osio-Vale * Craig Otterness *
Maura oude Lohuis * Megan Paige Owens *
Katherine Elizabeth Owings * Chloe ('Chloe-bear') Anne Painter *
Eric ('EJ') V. Palmer, Jr. * Sheila Palmer * Zoe ('Dipsy') Lucy Palmer *
Charlie Joon Park * 'Baby Parke' * Emma Rose Molly Parke *
Lucy Kingston Parker * Austin Parks-Schoen * Morgan Rachael Parrotta *
Antonina Partyka * Nicholas David Pawico, II * Cody Lee Payne *
Abbie Leone Pennington * Harvey James Percival *
Rishi Viraj Peshawaria * Cameron James Pete * Essey Petros *
Jessica Lee Phillips * Loren Ava Picinich * Dahrian Pimentel *
Brad Pittman * Samantha Poloka * James (Cayden) Poole *
Marshall Daniel Mo Potter * Caris Juliette Pourbaix * Gilly Powell *
June Price * Olivia Faith Price * Jacob ('Baby Bear') Daniel Procter-Trick *
Ava Louise Provoost * Nicole ('CoaCoa') Monet Pruitt *
Tony ('Big Man') Allen Pruitt, Jr. * Emma Purk *
Jordon Scott Pyke * Callum Rhys Quinn * Brianna Rakowiecki *

Jacob Isaac Rappoport * Taylor Lee Reagan * Debbie Reedy-Voyles *
Joseph ('Little Man') Blaine Reese * Isabella ('Bella') Porras Rehorst *
Haley Reid * Elva Björg Egilsdóttir Reynisson * Char'lea Richardson *
Julie Rigby * Conner Riggs * Amber Elizabeth Rivera *
Derek Kolby ('Kolby Cheese') Roberson * Alec Daniel Roberts *
Jace Anthony Robertson * Ryan Rodgers *
Francisco ('Panchito') R. Rodriguez, Jr. *
Harmony Alexandria Rodriguez * Courtney Lynn Roehrick *
Claire Elizabeth Roland * Rachel ('Rachelee') Rollinson *
Anne Jaso Roman * Lindsey Anne Ronningen * Daniel Ross *
Noah Paul Rouse * Maximilian Rubenstein * Sadie Russ *
Bradley ('Bobo') Steven Robert Ryall * Holly Saldana *
Carriejo Marie Sanders * Skylar Elizabeth Saranchuk * Anjali Sardar *
Elizabeth (Morgan) Saville *
Oscar ('Oscii Boscii Tchaikovsky') Finn Scallan-Cotter *
Claire Patricia Schafer * Jarred Kainalu Schaper *
Abbigail ('Abby') Elizabeth Marie Scheiderer *
Charles ('Charlie') William Scheuerman * Giuseppe ('Joe') Schifitto *
Zane Suzanne Schmid * Kourtney ('Special K') Nicole Schmidt *
Jonah Tyler Schuda * Tyler Luke Schuda * Chyanne Scott *
Noah Scott (BVVL) * Sheridan Scott * Thisbe Scott (BVVL) *
Kassidy Jade Sears * Elizabeth Semple * Matthew Sereni *
Debbie Shallow * Madelyn Grace Shannon * Cambell Jack Sheets *
Kayla Leigh Sheets * Grant ('Little G-Man') Thomas Sheppard *
Noah Shinn * Cameron ('Angel Baby') Lilly Shish * Michael Shoner *
Rachel Shoner * Owen Vincent Shuler * Audrey Nicole Shutes *
Erika ('Funny Girl') Nicole Silverthorne * Joliah Simmons *
Owen Reid Simmons *
Hannah Caitlin Simpson ('Our Angel with the Golden Glow') *
Ella ('Princess') Jade Sinclair * Glenn ('Glennie') Stewart Sinclair, III *
Julian George Oud Kendall Skelding * Christina Nicole Slack *
James Arlan Slattery * Eric Theodore Slavik * Jessica Anne Slavik *

Hailey Mae Smelser * Bradley Shane Smith * Bryan (Sawyer) Smith *
Cooper Jye Smith * Endia Smith * Ethan Douglas Smith *
Logan Michael Smith * Zachary Louis Span * Brian Thomas Spancake *
Truman James Spink * Gabriella ('Gabby') Yvette Stack *
Sarah Jane Staff * Devon Richard Stants * Sidney Houghton Stants *
Alyssa Gabrielle Stapleton * Sonja Natalia Stefanovic * Amanda Stein *
Lindsey Amber Stewart * Jordan Leo Stokes * Ryann Marie Stoll *
Matthew Tyler Storms * Jessica Nicole Stout * Wyatt Kyle Sutker *
Connor Swann * Cassidy ('Cassie') Swanson * Keira Sweeney *
David Alexander Swetz * Kaydence Deanna Tackett * Isaiah Ryan Taiwo *
Christopher ('Baby Chris') Nicholas Talley * Makayla Marie Tanner *
Alisha May Tansey * Elie Camille Tate * Hannah Lucille Tate *
Kassidy Jonette Tate * David Russell Tawn * Alex Krestensen Taylor *
Emmilee Victoria Tebeck * Katelyn Meredith Telley *
Arianna ('Ari') Ivon Tellez * Dakotah Storm Thornton *
Rosie Jane Tingey * Rachael Marie Tisdale * Sophia Victoria Torre *
Erin Trainor * Andrea Trakas * Jonathan Wade Tranby * Santie Truter *
Milos Turanjanin * Lisa Tyslan * Samantha ('Sam'/'Boopers') Jane Utzat *
Max Yorke Vallender * Katherine Mable ('Katie Mae') Vance *
Carl ('Carlo') Lawrence Vanderveen * Stijn van Houten *
Amanda ('Panders') Dawn Van Pelt * Leonardo ('Leo') Cobos Varela *
Mon Ami Vargas * Amanda Leigh Vaughan * Sanvi ('Naanoo') Vemula *
Maria Verdile * Madison Claire-Elizabeth Vickers *
James Matthew ('Matt') Vincent * Jessica Drew Vincent *
Leonardo ('Apepe') Volpi * Findlay Waghorn * Ms. Lam Ying Wai *
Master Leung Chin Wai * Janice Lenore Walden *
Virgil Freeman Walden * Maryclaire Elizabeth Walsh *
Christian Taylor Ward * Dynastie Unique Washington *
Logan ('Peanut') Watts * Cole Daniel Webb * Creg Kenyen Webb *
Timothy Weber * Josiah Steven Weiberg * Cynthia Carol Weingart *
Kayden ('Chunky Monkey') Faye Marie Wente *
Sierra Rose Wentworth * Anna Krystyna Werbowy * Piper Kier West *

Wayland Marshall West * Aiden Joseph White * Benjamin Jerrel White *
Samuel ('Sambob') Robert White * Mollie Carmel Whitfield *
Meghan ('Meggie') Emily Wiesner * Gabrielle Anais Wild *
Thomas Michael Wildes * William ('Will') E. Willardson *
Dallas McKenzie ('Kenzie') Willey * Hanna Reagan Willingham *
Piper Olivia Willingham * Dakota Reeann Willis *
Connie Lynn Palmes Wilson * Ronne Dartin Yondell Wilson *
Jordan Witzig * Sayre Matthew Wood * Courtney Jacob Woodard *
Tyler Matthew Woodard * Samantha Grace Woodson *
Kristin Lee Wormald * Kaitlin ('Katie') D. Wright *
Kristina ('Krissy') Wydela * Tysen Val Xavier * Nektarios Xirouxakis *
Xymhone John Roger * Alma ('Lil' Bun') Mae Yaeger * Amanda Yeater *
Tyler ('Our Little Angel') Yunes * Margaret ('Maggie') Zayas

♥ ♥ ♥

...to acknowledge a few of the countless others...

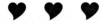

Ted * David * Catherine * Leah * Claire * Sofia * Addison *
Benjamin * Ali * Alexis * Jamie * Daniel * Alejandro * Joe * Abby *
Diana * Katie * Joseph * Janis * T. A. * Todd * Marvin * Talia * Kevin *
Delphine * Treven * Leah * Serena * Isabella * Agnés * Prudence *
Tara * Jose * Katherine * Luana * Tristan * A. A. * R. A. * B. A. *
Chastity * Eric * Tyler * O. A. * Al * Anthony * David * Seth *
Annette * M. B. * Charley * Chase * Chelsey * Jared * Rashad *
Anita * Peg * M. B. * Olivia * Sarah * Benjamin * G. B. * Jenica * Joe *
Charles * Carlene * Diana * Addison * Carolyn * Frank * Sasha *
Adam * Bill * S. B. * Beatriz * Sofia * John * Elizabeth * Jessica * Max *
Zachary * Lisa * Briahna * Allison * Megan * Ilsa * Chloe * Tom *
Kelly * Brendon * Michael * Madeline * Marco * Chrissy * Anita *

Van * Hannah * Kenneth * Kylee * Tom * Kevin * Heather * Matthew *
Steven * Eugene * Thomas * Kelly * Kris * Elva * Ethan * Jeremiah *
Kathryn * Becky * William * Christy * Chad * Sarah * Caitlyn *
S. B. * Lara * Kennedy * Maggy * Ethan * E. B. * Nick * Susan *
Jason * Jeremy * Lesa * Grant * Madison * Donna * Taylor *
Stephanie * Jeremy * Kristina * Breanna * Case * Michelle * Micheal *
Bethany * Elijah * Eugene * Jody * A. B. * Owen * Emily * Wayne *
Brooke * Celeste * Meghann * Camden * Mark * Amber * Seth *
Jadon * Jonathan * Zachary * Drew * Jonathan * Lenny * Mackenzie *
Tom * N. B. * Courtney * Barry * Landon * Madi * Virginia *
Richard * Sharon * Samantha * Elizabeth * Jennifer * Matt * Aubry *
Maggie * Brody * Kennedy * M. C. * Christa * Donna * Aaron *
Carolyn * Chase * Gavin * Kelly * Marie * Amanda * Anthony *
Anne * Tom * Garrett * Sarah * Brianna * Paige * Scott * C. T. C. *
Deven * Ben * Brittany * Brittany * Susan * Will * Jamey * Ethan *
Lauren * Emily * Bonnie * Katerina * D. C. * Liz * Sammy * Brandon *
Adyson * Santino * Annika * Benjamin * Matthew * Jenny * Jillian *
Celeste * Andrew * Larry * Shannon * Eric * Charlie * Brian * Ethan *
Kathryn * Sydney * Samuel * Luke * Chloe * Maria * Linda * D. C. *
Amy * Lucas * Grace * Rachel * Trisha * Ariana * John * Russ * F. C. *
Jamie * Kelsey * David * Diane * Jeffrey * Robin * Austin * Lucas *
Spencer * Jonathan * Joshua * Nathan * Jodi * Gary * Randy * George *
Kenneth * Michael * Joshua * Kelsey * Roberto * T. C. * Megan *
Robert * Bailey * Shonna * Jessica * Warren * Sophie * Josh * Emily *
Kelsi * C. L. C. * Kyle * Nicholas * Michael * Kevin * Zachary * Sue *
Molly * Jacqueline * Madison * Andrew * James * Laurie * Caroline *
Chris * Harvey * C-P. C. * Isabella * Anthony * Nicholas * Tess *
Hunter * Inna * Gracie * Christian * S. S. D. * Dan * Andrea *
Michael * Zoe * L. O. D. * Claire * Spencer * Carter * Samantha *
Evan * T. D. * Mariella * Grace * M.R.D. * Jessica * John * Santino *
Emily * Adam * John * Michele * Rebecca * Angela * Daryl *
Sharon * Kyle * Marcia * Rebecca * Dion * Zachary * Hunter *

Thayne * Alex * Henrique * Jordan * Katie * Erin * Ingrid * E. D. *
Sergio * Bob * Maria * Russ * Maria * Jessica * Doug * George *
Jacqueline * Joel * John * Mark * Jason * Dean * Kristen * Tammy *
Danita * Jack * Shayla * Aleah * Randy * Kristen * Tayler * Jolie *
Eric * Samantha * Theresa * Pablo * Katrina * Warren * Tanner *
Dean * Jason * Katie * Adam * Roy * John * Sofia * Hannah * Faith *
Charles * Y. E-S. * Ava * Melinda * Colton * Travis * Richard * Maria *
David * Andrew * Nathan * Dominick * Jack * Ellen * C. F. *
D. E. F. * Jake * Addison * Sara * Frankie * E. F. * Rita * Jan * Noah *
Wayne * Vanessa * Danny * J. F. * C. R. F. * Lynne * Zack * Marcel *
Jerry * Thomas * Kyle * E. F. * Sarah * Karla * Maggie * Steven *
Jack * SarahJane * S. M. F. * Nadine * N. F. * Devin * Kenton *
Lilee * Corinne * K. F. * Paul * S. F. * Christine * Conner * Natalie *
Matthew * Leo * Jessica * Kevin * Kyle * Anita * Ken * Christine *
Stephanie * Jenna * Alistair * Michelle * Andrea * Ethan * Madelyn *
Travis * Alejandro * Crystal * Tatiana * Allison * C. G. * Mat * Steven *
Tracee * Kris * Jack * Bruce * G. G. * Tomas * Gina * Nora * Micah *
Eric * Kylie * Cynthia * P. G. * Mary * Seth * Anna * Erin * Suzanne *
Dana * Matthew * L. G. * Burton * K. G. * Elena * Francisco *
Lorinda * J. J. G. * K. M. G. * Albert * Brian * Michael * O. G. *
Brandon * Michel * Katrina * Anna * Joel * Robert * Mike * Robert *
Nadia * Jim * Alice * Jack * Jonathan * Nicholas * Courtney * Luke *
T. G. * Gary * Lauren * Matthew * Rebekah * Sarah * Michael *
Jennifer * Jenna * Vivian * Z. G. * M. G. * Benjamin * Chad *
A. K. G. * G. G. * Ian * Debbie * Hannah * Laura * Isabella * Larry *
Tara * William * Jerry * Henry * Eric * Ethan * Courtney * Isabelle *
Charlene * Roberts * Dan *O. H. * Hallie * Woodrow * Arron *
Joshua * Isaac * Thomas * A. J. H.* Angel * Anita * Evan * Neal *
Ryan * Tyler * Charlie * Jack * Tammy * Jack * Savanna * Hannah *
Gregory * Jessica * Mikey * Z. H. * Meghan * Daniel * Danielle *
Stefanie * James * Hannah * Angelica * Jackson * Barbara * Robin *
Alexzandria * Meredith * Justin * Sarah * Claire * Robert * Peter *

Luke * Keith * Marci * Violeta * Andrew * Phillip * Madison * Laura *
Carly * Mason * Max * H. H. * Will * Blake * Katie * Matthew *
Jordyn * Philip * Amanda * Eddy * Jeff * Keith * Cody * Deborah *
Holly * Haley * Annie * Steve * Elaine * Joshua * Jennifer * Nathan *
Andrew * Selena * Abbey * David * Justin * Fanny * Carly * Brandy *
Annie * Charlie * Patricia * Bobby * Riley * Helena * Ann * Tyler *
Madelene * K. I. * Brigitte * Sam * Philip * Nathan * John *
Cassandra * Frances * Rachel * David * Jordon * Mary * William *
Cooper * Katie * Len * Ken * F. J. * Angela * Megan * S. J. * Edward *
S. B. J. * Briahnna * Colby * Derik * H. M. J. * Kyle * S. J. * William *
Andrew * Janet * Julie * Luke * M. J. * Paige * Richard * Royce *
Emma * A. J. * Tim * Abigail * Patrick * Troy * Rick * S. K. * I. K-I. *
Mona * Kevin * R. K. * T. K. * W. K. * Tony * Klara * Jack * Mary *
Donna * Ellyn * Jessica * Melissa * Marc * Daniel * Erin * Mal *
Douglas * David * Quintan * Gabriela * Owen * Pat * Camryn * Zoe *
Alexis * Zachary * Matthew * Ari * Gavin * Shane * G. K. * Destinee *
Liam * Brittney * W. K. * Nicholas * K. K-H. * J.. S. K. * Rosie *
Alivia * Brett * Joan * Jonathan * Robert * K. K. * K.. K. * K. K. *
Kent * Gavin * Susie * Jonathan * Trish * Leo * A. K. * Isabella *
Caroline * Bethany * Sarah * L. L. * Derek * William * Joseph * Julia *
Alexandra * R. L. * Penny * Chase * Amanda * Barry * Fernando *
Kelly * K. L. * H. L. * Blane * James * Nicholas * Anthony * Jennifer *
J. A. L. * Mary * Rebecca * Gerry * Marilyn * Abigail * Ryan * Chris *
Kathy * Patrick * Brian * Ruth * Jon * Gary * S-N. LeV-P. * G. L. *
L. N. L. * Randall * Sheridan * Gabrielle * Nathan * Joseph *
Jacqueline * Alvin * Shawn * Alice * J. L. * Jackson * George * Paul *
Kaitlyn * Nikolaus * Charlotte * Tyler * O. K. L. * Alicia * E. L. *
Jeff * Robbin * Lily * Kayleigh * Luke * Joseph * A. L. * Zachary *
Joseph * Melanie * Lucy * Colin * Meaghan * Grant * Camryn *
Mark * Hannah * T. A. M. * Andrew * Thomas * Angelo * Catarina *
Jenny * Connor * Eddie * Sam * Aaron * Daniel * Eric * Stephanie *
Tracy * James * F. M. * M. M. * Nicholas * B. M. * Jordan * Dan *

Daniel * Zachary * L. S. M. * Lewis * Ronald * Yves * Bella * Alexis *
Melissa * J. M. M. * Brooklyn * Theo * B. J. M. * Leslie * Alyson *
Nikolas * Pamela * Tina * Savannah * Mark * William * M. M. M. *
Colleen * J. J. M. * K. M. * Jake * Luke * Thomas * L. M. * Joseph *
Lisa * G. M. * Molly * Darren * Connor * Michele * Barry * Hugh *
Cody * Bonnie * Justice * David * Catherine * Jo * Luke * Meagan *
Natalie * Laura * F. M. * Alexandra * Victoria * Anthony * Rose *
Don * John * Spencer * Maxwell * G. M. * Christopher * Katherine *
C. M. * Angelo * Claudia * Dorien * Nathan * Jonathon * Michael *
Noah * Rosie * Ed * Tylar * Edward * S. M. * Toby * Brian * Floyd *
Joseph * K. T. M. * M. M. * Michelle * Natalie * Sally * Maya *
Virginia * Makenzie * S. M. * Maria * F. M. * Corey * Carly *
Kennedy * Nicole * Sarah * S. M. * Trisha * Monica * Ellie * Jake *
Toby * Kaiden * Nathan * Tanner * Jasmine * Tristan * Hannah *
Arden * Noah * E. S. M. * Christopher * Elisa * Celia * Caitlin *
Cody * Brianna * L. M. * Andrew * B. J. M. * M. J. M. * Michael *
N. S. N. * Nicole * Therese * Mikelle * Glenn * D. N. * A. N. * E. N. *
Bailey * Donna * Jessica * Laurie * Nicole * Quinn * Denny * Noelle *
Joan * Cody * Brian Joshua * Brenda * Ronald * Marina * G. N. *
Pamela * Kody * Kaitlyn * Owen * William * Deborah * Cooper *
Brad * Hailey * Mary * Peter * Randy * Conor * Chloe * Ginny * Pat *
Max * Brian * Jonathan * Tyler * Emily * Brenda * Armando * Joseph *
Mark * Natalie * Nathaniel * Jordan * Misty * Andrew * Matthew *
Celine * E. O. O. * P. O. * Fernando * Amanda * Julia * Alyssa *
Hannah * Matt * Elizabeth * Hannah * Robert * Mariana * M. P. *
Federica * Jeremiah * Anita P* Joan * T. P. * S. P. * R. P. * M. P. *
Joseph * Jill * Jamie * Connie * Desiree * Sean * Emily * Sharie *
Rebecca * Abbey * Eric * S. P. * Ian * Lisa * Adam * Jeremiah *
Danny * Stacy * Michal * Marco * Jack * Patrick * Christian * Hannah *
Christophe * Laura * Baylee * Ryan * Matthew * Shelby * Vincent *
Joshua * Michael * Christian * Harry * Eloise * Benjamin * Rob *
Robby * Colin * Alex * Brooke * Natalia * Joanna * Karen * Michael *

Nicholas * Sylvie * Arthur * Robby * Yvonne * Tomek * Ray * Aubrey *
Evie * Jacquelyn * John * Stephany * Alyssa * Alexandra * Erica *
Jean * Michael * Lisa * Jennifer * E. P. * A. A. Q. * J. M. Q. * Elyse *
Vern * Jalen * Zachary * Laurie * Oliver * Olivia * Chad * Madison *
Martin * Vanessa * Easton * Morgan * R. R. * Charles * James *
Kelly * S. R. * Brandon * Preston * Connor * D. R. * Timothy *
S. R. * Leah * Allison * Luke * Jennifer * Leandro * Garrett * James *
Becky * Kathryn * Colton * Brynne * Laura * Briana * Angeleena *
Scarlette * Pamela * Gray * Luke * Deirdre * Alfred * Danielle * Chris *
Theodore * C. R. * Thomas * Nicole * Taylor * Kennedy * Marley *
M. O. R. * Jose * Ryan * Shelby * Alexandra * Jake * Charles * Gary *
Dorothy * Larry * Stephanie * Jessica * Michael * Kyle * L. K. R. *
Reece * Corey * Connor * Scott * John * Brian * Robert * Sadie *
Colby * Ashton * Jacob * Liam * Matthew * Robert * John * Natalie *
Thomas * M. S-A. * M. S-A. * Michelle * Daniel * Gracee *
Constantine * Brianna * Sophia * Frank * Perez * Sarah * Rachel *
Isaih * Israel * Katherine * Z. S. * O. S. * V. E. S. * Emily * Benjamin *
B. J. * James * Kitty * Katie * Riley * Michael * Alexander * Brian *
Madeline * Michael * Russell * Abigal * Nathan * Penny * Quinn *
Austin * Samuel * Lee * Stephanie * A. R. S. * Emily * Nicholas *
Julia * Lindsay * Matt * Devan * Chris * Mark * Ivan * Matthew *
Andrea * Jessica * Santo * Lynne * Stephen * Greg * Ben * Owen *
Richard * Drew * Miranda * Andrew * Taylor * Logan * Hayley *
Kayley * Susan * C. P. S. * M. S. * Madison * Don * Thomas *
Brandon * Gary * N. S. * Y. S. * Valerie * S. R. S. * Lydia * P. S. *
Joshua * Marc * Danielle * Alyssa * Philip * Travis * Nick * C. S. *
Nathan * Thomas * Morgan * Ryan * Virginia * A. D. S. * Evan *
T. K. S. * Amy * Anne * Christian * Derek * Greg * Jason * Jerimiah *
Jessica * Julianne * Seth * Stuart * Vicky * Tina * Audrey * Ian * Julita *
Macarthur * Vanessa * Alfonsina * Cathi * Maria * Carole * Sadie *
Robert * J. D. S. * Y. S. * Noah * Jordan * Amber * Rachel * Brandon *
Mike * Dillon * Ashleigh * Diane * Jordan * Lisa * Katelyn * Becky *

Linda * Matthew * Craig * Ebony * Elizabeth * Kaitlyn * R. S. *
Rachel * Myles * Ellie * Dan * Keely * Dylan * Megan * Dillon *
Josiah * Adam * David * V. S. * Dale * T. S. * Jack * Justin * Madelyn *
Matthew * Kristina * N. M. T. * Donna * Darrius * Thomas * Daryl *
Jay * Cora * Emma * Marla * Darren * Tommy * C. T. * Billy *
Pierre * David * Owen * Paul * Danielle * Josephine * L. K. T. * Ross *
Tyler * Sebastian * Gage * Luke * Daniela * Jessica * Abbie * Katie *
Ashley * Carol * Heather * Jessie * Susan * Jeremy * Joshua * Cade *
Joy * Makayla * Michael * Rhylee * Todd * Terrell * Alexander *
Joshua * Greg * Hugo * P. T. * Joan * Anthony * Matthew * Isabella *
H. T. * Scott * Serena * Dominic * Victoria * Aaron * Terrence * E. T. *
Matthew * Harvey * John * Shane * Gary * Jean * Michael * Caden *
Andy * Kane * L. A. U. * K. U. * Luisa * R. T. V. * Desiree * Brent *
Hann * Rachel * Cynthia * Alicia * Lucas * Phillip * V. V. * Sean *
Eric * Evan * N. V. * Micheala * Alexis * Camille * Charlie * Emma *
Mike * David * Tyler * T. V. * Erina * Jonathan * Kathryn * Terry *
Dan * Seth * Hiliary * Tyler * N. W. * Shauna * Jenny * Keith * Hailey *
Hazel * Michael * Charlene * Crystal * Jared * Laura * Amos * Stewart *
Aimee * Amy * Linsey * Jonathan * Denise * Hailey * George *
Brooklyn * David * Jill * Ian * Lauren * John * Michele * Connor *
Hailey * Iris * P. W. * Craig * Emma * McKenzie * Ronald * S. W. *
Zach * Craig * Brittany * Jason * Laurie * Murray * Ronald * S. W. *
Autumn * Irene * Matthias * Jim * Kaiden * Carol * Michael * Taylor *
Audrey * Tori * Anna * F. W. * Amy * Ashley * Claudia * Larry * Emily *
Mark * Amelia * Buck * Haley * Jocelyn * John * Judy * Angela *
Georgia * Niki * Rhianna * Elias * K. M. Y. * Nathan * Carl * M. Y. *
B. S. Y. * Margaret * Casey * N. Y. * Liam * Hillary * N. Z. * Valentino *
Jeff * Mandi * Thomas * P. Z. * Y. R. Z. * Linzey * Corinna * Ian

About the Author...

Helen Baldwin and her husband, Randy, both originally from Fort Worth, Texas, live in the mountains of North Carolina, with occasional guest appearances by their college offspring. Randy is a high school health/physical education teacher and whiz of a football coach. He's also amazingly proficient in the areas of cooking and construction, and he's become quite proficient at waterfalls. However, one of his most stupendous achievements was his plunge from legitimate computer illiteracy to mastering complicated football software and figuring out how to do elaborate football DVDs for training, scouting, and entertainment. After enduring the miracle of that process, which included Randy's sending his very first email (of three), Helen retains hope that winning the lottery is still a possibility.

Their son, Matthew, graduates in the spring of 2010 with a master's in education on the same day their daughter, Katie, graduates (elsewhere, of course) with a major in photography. Jeffrey's spirited presence is everywhere.

Add a stubborn lab, goofy retriever, C-A-T, pond critters, and assorted wildlife to the typical challenges of an old farmhouse in a serene, rural mountain setting, and life stays entertaining in its own way. Their simple but inspirational surroundings encouraged them to add a small cabin, which is available for rental (shameless plug here, with more info at *angel-mountaincabin.com*).

Helen is the daughter of an elementary school teacher and principal, the late Elton Derden, and a retired piano teacher and extraordinarily gifted composer, JoAnn. Her brother, Paul, a physician, co-founded Crossroads Medical Mission (*crossroadsmedicalmission.org*), a mobile medical unit for underserved families in the rural crannies of southwest Virginia and northeast Tennessee. Paul is married to Jaymie, an exceptional dynamo in children's ministry programs and eager community volunteer. Their son, Jonathan, is a pilot, and their daughter, Bethany, is set to graduate alongside cousin Katie with a degree in psychology. She must figure she has plenty of subjects readily available.

For several years in a previous life, Helen taught young children with orthopedic and multiple handicaps in Columbia, South Carolina. She then retired happily to the status of 'just a mom.' Ha.

Not overly fond of writing until she quit being graded, Helen handled newsletter duties for the family's former lodge and collaborated with her mother, JoAnn, on <u>Tips for Making Music Fun & Easy!</u> as part of their work with the Smart Start program in North Carolina. <u>Tips </u>will undergo a mini makeover and be released again at some point.

Stepping way outside her comfort zone, Helen finally accepted primary responsibility for her own websites, keeping brudder Paul on speed dial for whatever she perceives as an emergency. She is most grateful that Paul's doctor skills, including compassion and patience for the less smart experienced, extend to tech stuff.

Thanks to a moment or two of insanity, Helen and Cindy Schaefer, good friend, fellow SMA mom, and Foreword writer, have dived collective nutty heads first into the world of blogging. The primary focus is on SMA matters, with a steady dose of 'normal' madness tossed in. If you dare, visit thesuitelifeoflucyandethel.blogspot.com.

<u>The Jeffrey Journey</u> is Helen's first solo book.

About the Composer...
(*Dreams for Jeffrey* CD available at thejeffreyjourney.com)

JoAnn Derden, the author's mother, received her classical training as a pianist at the Fort Worth Conservatory of Music, North Texas State University, and Texas Christian University. She enjoyed her many years of teaching and public performance, but a favorite pastime was always just 'making stuff up.'

With the incredibly advanced technology of keyboards and recording equipment, JoAnn has finally realized that she wants to continue doing just that 'when she grows up,' taking advantage of her fancy keyboard—a Korg O1W ProX Music Workstation. She says it makes her sound better than she really is, which makes it even more fun!

She has recorded several other albums, but *Dreams for Jeffrey* is one of the closest to her heart. While her inspiration for this album was her very special infant grandson, the tunes are soothing for souls of all ages. Be sure to read her verses accompanying the CD (p. 267)!

JoAnn and Elton, who remained her favorite critic even after 53 years of marriage(!), moved down the road from Helen and her family in the mountains of North Carolina only a few short months before Elton ('Papa') passed away. Confidence abounds, though, that he is still enjoying her music as much as the rest of the family; with his spirited inspiration, JoAnn has produced some of her best work ever!

Her latest release, truly inspired from Above, is entitled *Grief: Loss and Recovery*. It is a masterpiece, particularly powerful when it's realized that she just sits down and starts playing. It is currently available thru *thejeffreyjourney.com* and will gradually be joined by other CDs of her original compositions.

About the Other Contributors...

Ravelle Whitener graduated from Randolph-Macon Woman's College, where she studied art and computer programming and majored in dance. Years later, during some time 'off' to care for twin sons, Robert and Adam, she and Helen met and co-coached Odyssey of the Mind, where creative wackiness flowed effortlessly. She then started her own commercial art business, setting it aside to deal with the immediate success of a plastic films manufacturing company she and her husband, Rob, founded.

They were in the process of selling the company and envisioning a little free time when Helen burst that bubble with news of the original book and a desire for Ravelle to work her magic on the cover. Well, okay, Helen may have begged just a little. While Ravelle is not one to gloat over her work (which includes *A Tiny Angel*), Helen will happily gloat for her. Her contributions on The Jeffrey Journey have been simply perfect.

With this project completed, Ravelle was eager to renew some old interests... until all the boys in the family took up race car driving, requiring her to don her photographer's hat for a while. When that stint ended, Ravelle could think of nothing better to do than to renovate their lake house and move the family.

With an unlisted phone number.

∿

Katie Baldwin, the author's daughter and illustrator, has possessed unmatched wit and more than a few glimmers of creative genius since, well, birth. She was almost always a step ahead of her mom and provided spunk of some sort every day (there may—or may not—be a correlation between spunk and someone else's gray hair). She is on the brink of a college diploma (photography) and looking forward to seeing and shooting the world... and earning a living while doing it. She could not have been a better big sister to Jeffrey, although Matthew might balk at her *little* sister skills in the early days...

Bethany Derden, Helen's niece, has excelled in all endeavors, also since birth (these gals are something else)! She was a wonderful cousin to Jeffrey, doting on him as much as possible from her home two hours away. Her decision to write of her memories of him (*I Remember Jeffrey*) was encouraged and welcomed. Like Katie, she is a college senior, quite adept at photography (particularly babies and children!) but majoring in psychology... like her favorite mountainbilly aunt.

Watch out, world. These two are comin' through.

Dreams for Jeffrey
CD of lullabies by JoAnn Derden

1. Close My Eyes
Close my eyes... I'm dreaming
Sweet dreams that never end.

2. When My Mama Sings to Me
My very favorite time of all
Is when my mama sings to me.

3. I Love You, I Love You, I Love You, I Do!
Always know this I tell you is true–
I love you, I love you, I love you, I do!

4. The People Who Love Me
If I could, I would count
all the people who love me.
If I could, I would tell them
that I love them, too.

5. When Matthew Smiles
The world lights up when Matthew smiles–
More so than any other.
He smiles at me and makes me laugh–
I'm happy he's my brother!

6. Bethany's Green Eyes
Bethany's green eyes, green as the sea–
I feel so enchanted when she looks at me!

7. Jonathan's One-Man Band
The oboes, tubas, guitars sound so grand–
It's my cousin Jonathan's one-man band!

8. Mama and Daddy
My mama and daddy, the best that can be–
Thank you, dear Lord, for giving them to me.

9. The Cradle My Daddy Made for Me
Back and forth and back and forth,
I'm in my cradle Daddy made for me;
Left to right and back again,
Rocked in my cradle he made just for me.

10. Just Dreamin' 'bout My Mama
I'm just dreamin' 'bout my mama
If I smile while I'm asleep.
I'm happy when she cuddles me
And close to me she keeps.

11. Fast Asleep!
Off to dreamland!

12. Night Sounds on My Mountain
I love my little mountain–
On top you touch the stars.
At night it whispers songs to me
And secrets from afar.

13. Dreams for Jeffrey
I have the sweetest dreams on earth
All sugar, smiles, and songs–
Not just with me when I sleep,
They're with me all day long!

14. Playing with Katie's Hair
Softest brown with threads of gold
Her braids move with the air–
My fingers never touched more fine
Than through my Katie's hair!

15. Softly, Softly, in My Sweet Mama's Arms
Snuggled up in cotton clouds
Away from any harm,
I'm nestled where I love to be—
Right in my mama's arms.

16. God Bless My Friends and Family
Here is my prayer before I go—
God bless my friends and family,
And if there is a blessing left,
Thank You, God, for blessing me.

17. Angels Watching Over Me
Angel eyes are watching me,
Every night they sit—
Their golden lights surround my head,
Making sure my halo fits!

18. Kissing Me Goodnight!
Telling me goodnight and giving me a kiss,
Kissing me goodnight, and loving me...
All the way to dreamland.

19. Paul's Song for Jeffrey*
When I close my eyes
and am fast asleep,
I hear heavenly voices—
God's angels from the sky.
Stars so bright above—
filled with joy and love!
Angels calling Jeffrey...
Time to say good-bye.

*Paul, Jeffrey's uncle (and Helen's brother), came up with the melody, which JoAnn then transformed into a sweetly haunting expression of Jeffrey's farewell earthly dream...

Dreams for Jeffrey is available at thejeffreyjourney.com

Final Thoughts...

Beautiful. Wondrous. Enlightening. Uplifting. Sad. Wow—
it took me so many places, but left me feeling good. The music is
a wonderful complement. Both of these were the kind of things
the whole world needs to see, but only a select few will really
understand.

My job and my life in general force me to deal with death all
too often. This book will fortify me to deal with it and the folks
left behind. Thanks…

Your sweet Jeffrey was sent to you for a special purpose and
you have exceeded all expectations of what could come good of
it. Parents of any disabled child can identify with your moments
of horror and seeing that there can be someone who, at times,
sees that humor is a gift from God. None of us are fully prepared
for what life is going to bring us, but accepting it with grace,
compassion, humor and just flat accepting it is wonderful. What
you offer is hope. We all need that!!!! The many lives you have
touched are better for your having been there.

Mary Wooldridge, RN
(Nurse at former Brockman School)

Your book *The Jeffrey Journey* was truly the best Christmas
gift I have ever received. I felt as though I was reliving my own
story with someone who finally knew what it was like in receiving such a diagnosis.

I truly enjoyed the humor you brought to something so devastating and it gave me tremendous strength…

Jennifer Bolen, SMA parent

I just finished *The Jeffrey Journey*... The first 2/3 of the book were a frightening relapse of what Tisha and I went through just 8 short months earlier, and I was having a hard time reliving it but was curious to see how another family dealt with the sheer destruction SMA delivers the last months of a child's life. Your decision as a nurse and mother I could not support any better and I know that Jeffrey and Taylor are shining down on us.

We are planning on circulating the book, first throughout our family, having everyone sign the copy and leave a blessing for Taylor, then to close friends. In addition I plan to post a book review encouraging everyone to read *The Jeffrey Journey*.

Scott Reagan, SMA 'angel' parent

...it was really quite an experience to sit down and hold a book in my hands that was about SMA and a family dealing with it, it felt so RIGHT, you know? I don't know if saying I 'enjoyed' the book is the right phrase because of the content, although I did. But I appreciated it and recognized it and it touched me as I'm sure it will anyone who reads it...

Laura Stants, SMA 'angel' parent
Founder, SMA Support—www.smasupport.com

I read your book. I delayed for awhile because it's hard to read about someone losing their child. Especially, so shortly after Lindsey's death. However, I found it inspiring and a very compelling read. I was moved by your faith in God and your ability to see His work and His love in Jeffrey...

Thanks for having the courage to write such a book.

Brian Ronningen, SMA (self) and 'angel' uncle

This is one of the most well written books about a family and a crisis and all the struggles to get through it! We related to the story because we watched our daughter go through this with our grandson, Tommy! Rest in Peace, Tommy, Jeffrey, and all the other angels who left us. Cure SMA!

Kathie Harris, SMA parent

You have inspired me so much. I received your book Friday in the mail and never left the couch yesterday. I read the entire book in one sitting. I just couldn't put it down!

I must say, reading your book was like looking in a mirror. I too am a teacher, but of regular ed children. I used to look at special ed teachers and say, "Wow, I just could never do that. It takes a special person to handle those kids." I learned quickly, never say never. When things like SMA happen to people/children, you think… that happens to other people. How naive I was! I learned very quickly, I AM other people!

Reading your book has given me such a sisterly bond towards you. None of my friends truly understand how I feel or what I went through day to day.

I have never expressed the feeling of relief to anyone because it just does not sound right coming from a mother's mouth who lost her child. But the way you expressed it in your book… well it was perfect. You are an earth angel…

Courtney West, SMA 'angel' parent

I kept meaning to write you after reading the book to let you know how touched I was by it. I must've cried a river. I'd love to offer some profound words of how inspirational you and your family are, but I can't describe it. Most of all though, I found myself praying that your other two kids have grown up to be happy, healthy and well-adjusted *(note from Helen—they have!)*. I was so touched by their tenderness towards their little brother that I thought about them for days after reading the book…

Brenda Shofner, SMA aunt

…Through one of my other readers, I met Helen Baldwin, who has also gone through the heartbreak of losing a child. Helen sent me her book, *The Jeffrey Journey*. My heart broke with her. The two good-byes I've had with my two children were quick, with no time to prepare. It was not an agonizing, watching your child die before you, death.

At six weeks, Helen had that gut nagging feeling that something was wrong with her baby to the point of making her sick, which she called "ET"—extra terrified (I know that feeling.). At eight weeks of age, little Jeffrey was diagnosed with Spinal Muscular Atrophy (SMA). He had the most severe type called Werdnig-Hoffmann or Type I. SMA is the number one genetic killer for children under the age of two.

This book is Jeffrey's journey and their family's journey. Helen is blunt with what she goes through. She shares the notes she kept and the fight to keep her son alive. She questions her assignment from God. She fights to learn about the disease, and does not always just go along with protocol.

There is hope. Little Jeffrey's life has not gone in vain as this mom shares his story—their story. His life was worth fighting for. At the end Helen writes a letter to our Heavenly Father… a glimpse of why Jeffrey and ALL babies are worth fighting for…

If you or someone you know is or has fought a battle for a child, this is a must read book…

Loni Froehlich VanderStel, writingcanvas.wordpress.com

I just finished *The Jeffrey Journey*. "Thank you" is not adequate enough for putting your life, my life, to words; but "Thank you" is all I have right now…

Heather Kennedy, SMA 'angel' parent

I finally had the courage to begin reading your book last night and am so impressed. First of all it is wonderfully written, and I admire your sense of humor. Sometimes that is the only thing that gets us through the tough times. I can relate so much to what you went through even though the types between Jeffrey and Ethan are different—denial that there is anything wrong while really deep down knowing that there is, doctors, testing, poking, prodding, questions, financial concerns... It is hard to find others that understand because they haven't been through it...

Steph Och, SMA parent

...You wrote your story beautifully, and so much of it was so familiar. The pictures on the book made me want to look through your entire photo album—Jeffrey's beauty just shines through and it's so clear that he is beloved. Such little princes we had. I loved seeing Duncan's name in the dedication and all the other beautiful names—what a bond we all share...

Jeanne Jones, SMA 'angel' parent

I FINALLY got to read the book... I was able to read it in one sitting. Very easy to read and you captured the audience to want to keep reading. All I can say is, I had tears flowing several times. It is a beautiful story and tribute to an amazing little boy and his wonderful family. Everyone should read this and learn about how precious life is.

Annette Reed, SMA parent
Founder, Miracle for Madison and Friends
www.miracleformadison.org

The CD is beautiful, it is so peaceful, soothing and just wonderful listening...

Nancy Moore, SMA grandmother

...THE BOOK. It is fantastic. I have been trying to think of the right adjectives and they haven't come to me yet. One of my big impressions is what a gift this will be for so many people. It is a huge contribution—one of those things that will have tremendous and far-reaching effects that you will never even be able to imagine, but must trust are there. It will undoubtedly help in the quest to overcome SMA. It will surely give comfort to MANY whose hearts have been broken by various life events (what an incredible contribution to humanity!). It is simple, in some ways, but HUGE—by sharing this, you will make quite a ripple in the lives of many. It would be my dream to leave such a legacy in life.

Reading it was both fascinating and WRENCHING. The profits of the Kleenex manufacturer (or rather their cheap competitors) will soar after my trip through the pages. And yet, after I had finished every single page (I even read EVERY name), I was surprised by a wonderful sense of calm. I thought that was so interesting in light of the peace you described after Jeffrey became an official angel.

I've decided that if anyone can read this without being strongly moved, we will promptly ship them off to med school and arrange for them to go into partnership with Dr. Usually-Right.

Leckie Conners, friend

For more information about The Jeffrey Journey, visit thejeffreyjourney.com

A portion of the profits from the sale of <u>The Jeffrey Journey</u>
is designated for SMA research and/or
the myriad needs of families.

LaVergne, TN USA
22 March 2010

176730LV00008B/3/P